The Hypericum Handbook

The Hypericum Handbook

USING ST. JOHN'S WORT, ''NATURE'S PROZAC,''

TO ALLEVIATE DEPRESSION

Carol A. Turkington

M. Evans and Company, Inc.
New York

M. Evans and Company, Inc.
216 East 49th St.
New York, NY 10017

Text design by Leah Lococo

ISBN 0-87131-857-1

Printed and bound in the United States of America

Trade Paperback Edition

9 8 7 6 5 4 3 2 1

For Marianne Burkholder

Contents

Appendices

Introduction

For more than 2,000 years, depressed patients have turned to a rangy yellow weed known as hypericum, or St. John's wort, to treat the symptoms of unrelenting sadness. So powerful is this medicinal herb that ancient healers believed hypericum not only vanquished depression but was effective against the Powers of Darkness as well. It was said the herb was so obnoxious to evil spirits that even a brief sniff would banish them forever to the underworld.

Today, more and more people believe that the herb, also known as St. John's wort, still carries significant power—at least when it comes to depression. Nature's answer to Prozac has been attracting supporters around the globe as more and more mainstream scientists are discovering that it works as well as certain antidepressants without the harmful side effects or the high cost. In Germany alone, physicians write 3 million prescriptions a year for St. John's wort—more than 25 times the number for Prozac.

Europeans have historically been more open to herbal medicine, but more recently scientists in the United States also have begun to take an interest in the antidepressive qualities of St. John's wort. No less an authority than the *Journal of Geriatric Psychiatry and Neurology* devoted an entire issue—with 17 research papers—to hypericum. In another review of 23 controlled studies involving 1,757 depressed patients published in the *British Medical Journal*, scientists reported that St. John's wort worked three times better than a placebo in relieving depression, and equally as well as several prescription antidepressants.

It's the herb's surprising lack of side effects that makes it so intriguing, according to Purdue University herbal expert Varro Tyler, M.D. The problem with modern antidepressant drugs is that all of them carry significant risk of side effects, including serious sexual dysfunction and even death when used inappropriately. "The absence of serious side effects [with St. John's wort]," according to Tyler, "is one of its biggest selling points."

The need for a low-cost antidepressant that is widely available and carries few side effects is critically important in a country like the United States, where 2 out of every 10 Americans live their lives teetering on the brink of depression, without any expectation that things will improve. As many as 23 percent of all women have had one major depressive episode in their lifetime.

Those who have had one episode of depression have a 50 percent chance of having another bout—sometimes four or five episodes during a lifetime. Yet while so many people struggle silently with their misery, few ever seek professional help. Of the 18 million Americans who are depressed, 12 million today are not getting any treatment at all.

One of the main reasons many people hesitate to get help is that they are reluctant to take antidepressants, usually because people have heard frightening stories of side effects, or because they understand that it can take a long time to find the right drug. Others simply can't afford the high cost of antidepressants. In a country that still views depression not as a disease but as a moral weakness, many fear the social stigma of taking prescription drugs to treat depression. For these reasons, a natural alternative to antidepressants holds much appeal. If you are eager to learn alternative ways of easing your symptoms, *The Hypericum Handbook* can provide those answers.

ATTENTION!

The Hypericum Handbook is not intended to prescribe or diagnose in any way, nor is it meant to be a substitute for professional help. The information in this book is general and is not specific to individuals and their particular circumstances. Any plant, whether used as food or medicine, externally or internally, can cause an allergic reaction in some people.

Readers should not self-diagnose or self-treat for any serious or long-standing problem without consulting a medical professional or qualified practitioner. Always seek medical advice if symptoms persist.

If you are already taking any antidepressant, don't change your dose or combine it with hypericum without talking to your doctor first. This is particularly true if you are taking any MAO inhibitor (see Chapter 6). You should also see your doctor if you have any type of pre-existing medical condition or psychiatric disorder.

IF YOU ARE THINKING OF SUICIDE

If you are having suicidal thoughts—if you think there is the slightest chance you may act on your suicidal thoughts—get emergency help at once. Don't rely on treating yourself with St. John's wort—or anything else.

- Call 911.
- Call a suicide hotline.
- Call your doctor.
- Call your religious counselor.

As many people know, suicidal thoughts are often a part of depression. Thinking about *acting* on these thoughts is a danger sign. You need to get help at once.

CHAPTER 1

Depression

Everybody feels a little sad sometimes. In some circumstances, it may even be *appropriate* to be depressed, as Ellen McGrath, Ph.D., describes so eloquently in her book *When Feeling Bad Is Good* (Bantam Books, 1992).

The main difference between "the blues" and a true depression is that your sad feelings lift after a day or two. A major depression is far more persistent: It's been described by sufferers as "a gray drizzle of horror," a "dark cloud," a "numbing pain." People who are depressed often feel that their bleak outlook will never improve. The feelings may interfere with sleep, appetite, sexual interest, self-image, or attitude. (For an "Are you depressed?" quiz, see Appendix G.) The dreadful feeling can last for weeks, months—or years.

This chronic, progressive disease may oddly enough be hard for many people to diagnose in themselves. You may be depressed, and then go into remission, and then become depressed again. Chances are that—without treatment—depression will strike again and again, more quickly and powerfully each time.

It's an illness, not a moral weakness, and it affects more than 17 million adult Americans each year and costs the nation up to $44 billion in treatment, disability, and lost productivity. The illness, often chronic or recurrent, affects mood, thoughts, body, and behavior.

TYPES OF DEPRESSION

Chronic Minor Depression

Known medically as "dysthymia," chronic minor depression can make you feel mildly depressed all the time—even for years on end. It used to be called "depressive neurosis" in the 1950s and "depressive personality" in the 1970s. This type of mild depression, which may affect as many as 3 million Americans at any one time, is one that responds extremely well to St. John's wort.

It can be important to treat minor depression, first because it's unpleasant, and second because it's possible that mild depression can lead to major depression. Treating the symptoms early can help head off this worsening of the condition.

Your doctor may diagnose dysthymia if you have been depressed during most of the past 2 years, with at least three of these symptoms:

- low self-esteem
- withdrawal
- fatigue
- lack of interest in former pleasure
- difficulty concentrating or making decisions
- irritability/excess anger
- low productivity
- pessimism
- hopelessness or despair

Subclinical Depression

Another type of mild depression that seems to respond very well to St. John's wort is subclinical depression. People with this problem may have only two or three symptoms of depression (see Appendix G) as opposed to five or more. If this is your case, odds are you've never sought mental health treatment for your low moods, since you can probably function fairly well despite your feelings of emptiness and fatigue.

Atypical Depression

Most depressed people don't sleep or eat enough—but it's possible to be depressed without having the typical symptoms. People with this problem—called atypical depression—often continually crave sleep, food, or sex over a period of at least 2 weeks. They may be anxious, and extremely sensitive to environment and rejection. Atypical depression may be disguised as bulimia, anorexia, compulsive overeating, oversleeping, addictions, or impulsiveness, and it's more common in women.

Major Depressive Disorder

Symptoms differ from one person to the next, but major depression is almost always characterized by general feelings of sadness and a complete loss of pleasure in things that once brought you joy. There may be sleep problems, eating issues, a sense of worthlessness, or complete loss of interest in sex. A typical episode of a major depressive disorder, according to the *Diagnostic and Statistical Manual of Mental Disorders*, lasts at least 2 weeks and includes most of the symptoms listed in Appendix G. You need to understand that if you've had one major episode of depression, you've got a 50 percent chance of having another bout (maybe four or five bouts in a lifetime).

Of course, it is possible to have a major depression and not feel especially sad or hurting. You may just have eating problems, sleeping problems, or problems remembering, concentrating, or making decisions. Only a mental health expert can diagnose your depression and decide whether you have mild or moderate depression, which would be appropriate for St. John's wort, or whether you have a severe depression, which should be treated with antidepressants.

Other Types of Depression

Experts emphasize that St. John's wort is *not* recommended for certain types of depression. These include people who are severely depressed, who may have suicidal thoughts, or who have manic-depression (bipolar disorder). People with psychotic depression (characterized by hallucinations, delusions of guilt, serious medical illness, and so on) are not good candidates for hypericum either.

SPECIAL PROBLEMS OF DEPRESSION

Women and Depression

It's a fact of modern-day America: More than twice as many women as men are diagnosed with depression. A shocking 1 out of every 4 women will experience a depressive episode sometime during her life. The reasons *why* are both controversial and elusive.

Some experts blame a woman's physiology, either hormone imbalances or heredity. Others say it's the different way women are taught to handle their emotions. Still others say it's that health experts are more ready to diagnose a depression in women. Lastly, some blame society—poverty, susceptibility to abuse, physical and sexual abuse, lower social status.

Careful studies have found that the high percentage of depression is *not* related to the fact that women are just more willing to say they are more depressed—in fact, they really *do* get depressed at a greater rate.

Children and Depression

While you may think of depression as a problem of adulthood, in fact it can appear as early as infancy. In one study of 3,000 children, almost 15 percent were depressed; by age 15, the number had increased to include 1 out of 5. Furthermore, most experts think that children who have had one episode of depression early in life are at risk for future episodes.

Yet the use of antidepressants in childhood is controversial, especially because of the unpleasant or serious side effects so many of these drugs have. While extensive studies of St. John's wort in children have not been done, the plant is generally considered mild and fairly harmless. Herbalists recommend that small doses be given to younger children who should be under the care of a health expert no matter what treatment is given. St. John's wort should not be given at all to children under age 2.

Popular culture may have us convinced that, by the time kids reach adolescence, depression in teenagers is a normal phase. In fact, while adolescence is certainly turbulent, there is no reason why teenagers should struggle with depression when treatment is available. In fact, it is critical that true depression should be treated at this age because of the high risk of suicide. St. John's wort, as a milder, gentler treatment, may be a good choice for some depressed teens, especially because of the low side effect profile.

Depression in the Elderly

Up to 20 percent of the more than 30 million senior citizens in this country may be depressed, but their feelings are too often misinterpreted or ignored. Because age carries such a negative connotation in the United States, there is an unspoken feeling that it just makes sense to be sad if you're old, since it's just an unpleasant time of life. In fact, depression should *not* be a normal part of aging, any more than it should be a normal part of adolescence. The fact that depression is four times more common in this age group, and that the suicide rate is very high, does not mean that depression should be acceptable or inevitable.

Still, it's easy to see how depression in the elderly can be overlooked. It's often misdiagnosed and confused with distractibility, indifference, memory loss, and senility. In fact, 12 percent of the elderly who are diagnosed with dementia are really just depressed. They may have Cushing's syndrome or Parkinson's disease, thyroid disease, pulmonary disorders, vitamin deficiencies, cancer, or stroke—all of which can be linked to depression.

Because metabolism slows with age, older people should use a smaller-than-average dose of St. John's wort. The plant is often a sensible choice because of the low risk of side effects, compared to traditional antidepressants which can be particularly bothersome for people over age 65.

CAUSES OF DEPRESSION

Most experts would agree that depression doesn't have one simple cause. Instead, it is probably caused by a complex interplay of chemical interactions and personal experience. The physiological basis of depression lies in the nerve cells within the brain. Those that are responsible for our emotions are embedded in a part of the brain called the hypothalamus, a structure about the size of an olive that controls hunger, thirst, sleep, sexual desire, and body temperature.

In order for anything within your body to get done, your cells have to communicate with each other. The cells in your brain communicate via neurotransmitters, sending messages across the gaps between cells. Each neurotransmitter has a special shape that works like a key to fit into a "receptor" on a neighboring cell, like a key in an ignition switch. When the neurotransmitter "key" is inserted into the receptor "ignition," the cell fires, and sends the message on its way. Then, once the message is sent, the neurotransmitter messenger is either absorbed into the cell or burned up by enzymes in the gaps.

When these neurotransmitter levels are unusually low, messages can't get from one cell to the next and communication in the brain slows down. Experts believe you may get depressed if the levels of some of the neurotransmitters are low, or if the neurotransmitters don't fit into the receptor "ignitions" for some reason.

There may be more than 100 different types of neurotransmitters, but those that seem to be most important in the feelings of depression include serotonin, norepinephrine, and dopamine. The pathways for these neurotransmitters can be found in the very parts of the brain that control functions that don't work well in depression—sleep, appetite, mood, and sexual interest.

But we don't know if depression is directly related to abnormal amounts of neurotransmitters, or whether these neurotransmitters affect other chemical processes in the brain that aren't yet understood. Still, it's clear that neurotransmitters are related to depression, since medications that boost the levels of these neurotransmitters also ease depression.

What's odd is that some of the newer antidepressants don't affect the levels of all these neurotransmitters, but they still relieve depression. Other substances (such as cocaine) that do interfere with neurotransmitter levels don't affect depression.

It appears that St. John's wort affects several different types of neurotransmitters all at once, in unique ways unlike any antidepressant drug. What really puzzles scientists is that antidepressants and St. John's wort all raise the neurotransmitter levels almost immediately—but your depression won't lift until weeks after treatment starts. This is why we think that depression is a far more complex problem than a simple low level of neurotransmitters. Depression is probably influenced by a complex interaction of receptor responses and neurotransmitter release, not just how many neurotransmitters there are, but how many and how effective the receptors are.

As scientists continue to study St. John's wort, they hope to find out how some of the more than 50 active compounds in the plant interact to influence brain chemistry in subtle ways—so that depression lifts *without* the unpleasant side effects caused by every synthetic antidepressant drug.

Life Events

Of course, there is more to depression than the simple chemical interactions in your brain. Depression can be triggered by a wide range of unpleasant life events, such as loss or trauma, hormonal events like PMS or pregnancy, endocrine disorders, heredity, drugs, and other influences such as body rhythms and the seasons.

Loss or trauma

Most of the time, it seems that a depressive episode can be set off by a significant loss or a trauma. In one twin study of 680 pairs, a life stress such as divorce or death was the best way to predict depression. It doesn't have to happen this way, though—depression can descend seemingly from out of nowhere.

Hormones

Depression, however, can be caused both by events outside the body and events within it. Hormones and depression are intricately linked, so that many women experience a depression whenever hormone levels fluctuate—at puberty, during PMS, during pregnancy, after birth, at perimenopause. This isn't surprising, since hormones affect the activity of neurotransmitters, which in turn affect the timing and release of hormones.

For this reason, St. John's wort has historically been used as a treatment for "women's problems" surrounding menstruation and menopause. A woman's cycle is regulated by the interaction between serotonin, dopamine, and norepinephrine, together with pituitary and ovarian hormones. A low level of serotonin, in particular, has been implicated in PMS—and it is serotonin that St. John's wort is known to balance.

It is hormones that affect up to 70 percent of new mothers, who often experience a mild form of depression, including crying spells and restlessness; symptoms often fade within a week. A much smaller number will develop true postpartum psychosis, turning rapidly from a mild depression to delusions and hallucinations. Of course, these symptoms are not the sort that should be treated by St. John's wort, but need to be referred to a qualified mental health expert.

Endocrine disorders

Several endocrine or hormonal diseases may cause depression, including underactive thyroid (hypothyroidism), overactive thyroid (hyperthyroidism), Addison's disease (underactive adrenal gland), Cushing's syndrome (overactive adrenal gland), and abnormalities of the parathyroid gland. Hormonal drugs (birth control pills, cortisone, or prednisone) also may lead to depression.

Inherited depression

Doctors aren't sure whether there is a single "depression gene," but it certainly seems clear that the tendency to develop depression can run in families. This is particularly true for manic-depression; at least half of all manic-depressives have at least one parent with the disorder. (For more information on your chances of inheriting depression, see Appendix I.)

Rather than a single gene, you probably inherit the tendency to depression both from a range of genes and from personality traits that may be known collectively as a "depressive personality disorder." People with the disorder tend to brood, fuss, and be overly critical of others and themselves. Some people with a depression problem are born with a different type of brain biochemical makeup, with personally high levels of stress hormones and low levels of "calming neurotransmitters" like serotonin and norepinephrine.

Depression-causing drugs

Many drugs now on the market may inadvertently cause depression. These include Catapres, Aldomet, Inderal, drugs used to treat Parkinson's disease (such as L-dopa), diet pills, and medicines prescribed for arthritis, ulcers, and seizures; and hormones like estrogen, progesterone, and cortisol. Rarely, some tranquilizers (such as Valium or Halcion) can set off a depression. (See Appendix J.)

Other influences

Depression can also be influenced by your body's natural rhythms, and by the seasons. Your body's internal clock governs almost everything that happens in your body, including temperature, hormone secretion, and sleep-wake patterns. These so-called circadian rhythms may affect your depression, too—you may feel better at one time of day than another. Some people appear to have a malfunctioning clock that makes them vulnerable to seasonal affective disorder (SAD), or "winter depression." As many as 35 million Americans may suffer from this problem—some estimates suggest up to half of all women in northern states may have the winter blues. It is believed to be related to the pineal gland, melatonin, and a lack of natural light.

SAD is often treated by having the depressed person sit under special lights each day. Recently, doctors are turning to substances that work on the serotonin pathway—including Prozac, similar antidepressant drugs, and St. John's wort—to treat SAD. However, **because of the possibility that St. John's wort can induce extreme sensitivity to the sun, it is important that people with SAD not use the plant together with light therapy.**

At the Doctor's

You stand the best chance of beating depression if you combine counseling with some type of medication—whether that is St. John's wort or a standard antidepressant. Research clearly shows that medication or herbs alone work less well; coupling them with "talk therapy" means you're treating all of the causes and the symptoms. Besides, you'll need to see a doctor anyway to get a prescription for antidepressants, and if you choose to take St. John's wort, you should be under a doctor's care as well.

When you arrive at the office, the doctor will probably begin with a brief family history, together with a medical workup. Your doctor will want to rule out many diseases that may cause depression, including an underactive thyroid, anemia, diabetes, adrenal insufficiency, or hepatitis. Your doctor will also want to know about any drugs you may be taking, since there are a number of prescription drugs that can cause depression (see Appendix J). You'll also want to include any vitamins, other herbal medicines, amino acids, diet supplements, or recreational drugs you may be taking.

Counseling Therapy

While St. John's wort for many people is a good alternative to antidepressant drugs, everyone who is depressed should also be seeing a counselor to talk about depressed feelings. There are a range of different types of therapy, however. You may be more comfortable with one than another.

Cognitive therapy is based on the idea that depression is caused by a distorted way of thinking—that how you think affects how you feel. This type of therapy can identify problems with your ways of thinking that can cause depressive attitudes.

Behavior therapy teaches you how to change your distorted thoughts and alter your behavior. It's based on a system of self-rewards and can be especially helpful if you have phobias or panic attacks.

Interpersonal therapy emphasizes the development and improvement of relationships. Psychodynamic therapy is a lot like classical psychoanalysis, exploring your past for unresolved emotional conflict. Group therapy helps you learn about how to cope with your depression within a group of people who share similar problems and issues.

Lifestyle Changes

In addition to formal "talk therapy" and treatment, either with drugs or with St. John's wort, if you're depressed odds are you'll benefit from making some lifestyle changes, too. There's solid evidence that regular exercise, such as walking, running, or biking, can ease some moderate forms of depression by raising the level of certain mood chemicals in your brain—the same ones affected by St. John's wort. Think of exercise as *boosting* the effect of your St. John's wort therapy. You don't need to be an Olympic marathon runner to benefit— even a brisk 10- or 20-minute walk can help. However, exercise has not shown to be effective in easing a severe depression.

TYPES OF ANTIDEPRESSANTS

There are many types of depression, and many ways to treat it. The truth is, no single antidepressant or herb works for everyone. The good news, however, is that one of them will work for up to 80 percent of everyone with depression.

The good thing about St. John's wort is that it appears to combine many of the aspects of *different* classes of antidepressants in one natural substance. However, it's a good idea to have at least a general notion of other types of antidepressant drugs, because for some people St. John's wort just doesn't work. In that case, your doctor will need to work with you to find a medication that will.

How They Work

What St. John's wort and antidepressants have in common is that they all correct a chemical imbalance or dysfunction in the brains of depressed people. They all boost the level of at least one type of neurotransmitter in various ways. However, different drugs alter different systems.

There are several different classes of antidepressants: tricyclic antidepressants (TCAs), monoamine oxidase inhibitors (MAOIs), selective serotonin reuptake inhibitors (SSRIs), and other, structurally unrelated drugs (like Wellbutrin, Effexor, and Desyrel). TCAs, or tricyclics, boost the level of norepinephrine, epinephrine, serotonin, and dopamine by blocking their reabsorption. MAOIs destroy enzymes responsible for burning up neurotransmitters, which raise their levels. SSRIs interfere with the reabsorption of serotonin. Bupropion (Wellbutrin) affects dopamine; Effexor affects norepinephrine, serotonin, and dopamine; and Desyrel affects serotonin.

Your doctor will probably need to try several different combinations in order to find the one substance that will ease your depression. If several drugs haven't worked, you may want to try St. John's wort next. If St. John's wort doesn't work, you may want to move on to an antidepressant, and work your way down the list until you and your doctor find one that does work. The important thing is not to give up!

Side Effects

The main reason so many scientists are excited about St. John's wort is that the risk of side effects is low. Antidepressants carry a long laundry list of possibilities: sedation, dry mouth, blurry vision, constipation, urinary problems, increased heart rate, memory loss, dizziness on standing, tremor, sexual problems, movement disorders, endocrine system changes, stomach problems, insomnia, and anxiety.

Among this long list of problems, each drug has its own profile. Tricyclics often cause dry mouth, constipation, sedation, nervousness, weight gain, and diminished sex drive. MAOIs interact with certain foods and medications to produce potentially fatal high blood pressure. Newer SSRIs (like Prozac) can cause anxiety, nausea, headache, and sexual problems.

Blocking different neurotransmitters causes separate side effects; this is why the older drugs that blocked more than one neurotransmitter cause more problems. Yet St. John's wort, which appears to affect almost all neurotransmitters, causes no side effects. It's one of the paradoxes of the plant that have so far puzzled doctors.

SUICIDE

The primary risk of any depression is suicide. Anyone who has had or is having suicidal thoughts should not be taking St. John's wort, but should be under the care of a mental health expert and—most likely—taking antidepressant drugs. While St. John's wort appears to be enormously effective with mild and moderate depression, it has not been tested against more serious emotional problems. Because of this, experts are afraid that St. John's wort might not work against a serious depression, leaving the patient vulnerable to despair and suicide.

Since St. John's wort can take up to a month to become effective—longer than antidepressant drugs—a person at risk for suicide would be vulnerable for a long period of time. It is estimated that 30,000 Americans kill themselves each year, and at least 10 times that number make failed attempts. Suicide is a special problem among the young—five teenagers every day commit suicide in the United States. And for every teen who commits suicide, another 200 try. (See Appendix H for warning signs of potential suicide.)

CHAPTER 2

What is St. John's Wort?

St. John's wort is an ancient herb steeped in magic, mysticism, fairies, and rituals. Today, the rangy yellow weed called St. John's wort is making a reverential comeback as the herb to have—only this time, it's because of its apparent ability to heal depression.

Its reputation for possessing healing magic may have come in part from the plant's tendency to "bleed" a red juice when bruised. To ward off evil, the Germans hung it over their doorways, the pre-Christians stuffed it into amulets around their necks, and even St. Columba himself hid a branch of St. John's wort inside his robes. It was whispered that the plant could make warlocks fly, fend off thunderbolts, and avert the Evil Eye. Wielding a sprig of the plant, wise women whispered that you could predict a death or a wedding. And if you stepped on hypericum at twilight, the ancients believed you might be carried off on a magic fairy horse and not return until daylight.

The ancient Greeks heralded St. John's wort for its alleged magical powers as well. Its scientific name—*Hypericum*—comes from the Greek *Hyperieum*, meaning "over an apparition," a reference to the fact that this herb was so hated by evil spirits that a whiff of it would make them fly. Incantations were whispered over this herb when used as an amulet for protection in pre-Christian religious rites. Pagans would light huge bonfires with the plant—St. John's fires—and sing, dance, pray, and perform magical and symbolic ceremonies around the flames.

Its origins lost in the mists of antiquity, hypericum is believed to have been associated with the sun god Balder, because of its golden flowers and ray-like cluster of stamens. When pagan Balder's Day was transmuted by the Christian priests into St. John's Day, the plant's affiliation was likewise transferred to St. John as well.

The legends surrounding this herb are many and varied, and stories of the source of its name abound. No one knows for sure, but many authorities suspect that the plant's namesake most probably was John the Baptist. It is said to bloom on his birthday (June 24) and bleed red oil on the day in August when he was beheaded. Other stories suggest that the name may have come from the fact that the blackish-red spots on the petals of St. John's wort represent the blood shed by John at his beheading, and the translucent spots on the leaves represent the tears shed over that event.

Whatever the case, it is clear that by the sixth century A.D., according to the Gaels, the Christian monk St. Columba—who revered St. John—liked to tote a piece of the plant around in his robes for good luck. It was supposed to ward off evil spirits, especially when worn on St. John's Eve (June 23). Medieval peasants believed they could protect themselves against witches, warlocks, and the Evil Eye by bringing the flowers of St. John's wort into the house on Midsummer Eve.

And if you wanted to protect yourself from dying, according to the 1733 herb book *A New English Dispensatory*, you should sleep with a piece of the plant under your pillow on St. John's Eve. If you did this, the saint would "appear in a dream, give his blessing and prevent one from dying in the following year." It was traditionally gathered on one day only—St. John's Day—when it was soaked in olive oil to produce the blood-red anointing oil known as "the blood of Christ."

But what began as a magic herb was soon being used for medicinal purposes as well. For thousands of years, herbalists have used the plant not just for depression, but topically as a wound and burn healer, and orally as a remedy to treat a variety of viral and bacterial conditions. *Wort* is the Old English word meaning "healing herb." St. John was also the patron saint of nurses, and St. John's wort was known as "the healing herb for nurses." The ancient medical authorities Hippocrates (460–377 B.C.), Dioscorides (A.D. 41–68), Galen (A.D. 150–200), and Pliny (A.D. 23–79) all used St. John's wort as a medical treatment—usually for "women's complaints." In the Middle Ages, herbalists were prescribing it for depression and anxiety. By the mid–nineteenth century, the Shakers—master herbalists and mail-order entrepreneurs—sold St. John's wort as a cure for "low spirits."

To this day, you can hear references to the plant in American blues music, which mentions using "John de Conqueroo" (the root of the St. John's wort plant) to put a spell on enemies. Now it's putting a spell on the public, who are clamoring to buy this latest weapon in the war on depression. St. John's wort today is now the leading antidepressant in Germany, outselling Prozac 20 to 1. In fact, it outsells all other antidepressants combined. In the United States, sales have been taking off since autumn 1996 and have been steadily climbing ever since.

Description

St. John's wort includes any species of the large and widespread genus *Hypericum*, of the family Hypericaceae (St. John's wort family)—there are about 200 species in the family. It ranges in size from the tiny, 4-inch, matted *Hypericum anagalloides* (bog St. John's wort) to the tall *H. perforatum*, which can reach 32 inches tall.

Also known as the Fourth of July flower, St. John's wort blooms from early July through August in a variety of habitats, depending on the species. In general, the larger species are found in dry to moist open hillsides, up to 6,000 feet above sea level. The higher the elevation and the wetter the ground, the smaller the species. It can be seen in uncultivated woods, in hedges, along roadsides, and in meadows.

An Asiatic plant that was brought to this country via Europe, St. John's wort can be found throughout the Pacific and Rocky Mountain states as well as in more isolated areas in the central and eastern parts of North America. A species of hypericum is one of several plants called Aaron's beard, because of the beard-like look to its stamens. In the Pacific Northwest, *H. perforatum* and *H. formosum* are found profusely carpeting the open rangelands in the foothills. Here these species are considered noxious weeds and attacked with herbicides.

The plant used as an antidepressant—*H. perforatum*—is a sturdy perennial weed with yellow, five-petaled flowers topped by a burst of three stamen bundles. *Perforatum* comes from the Latin word for "perforated," referring to the leaves, which when held to the light reveal translucent dots that give the impression the leaf is perforated. The dots are not holes in the leaf, however, but a layer of colorless essential plant oils and resins. Many herbalists believe that the translucent perforations and the black-red spots contain the most active medicinal substances.

These small, oblong, opposite leaves, with each pair crossing those above and below, are usually light green and sprout from a stem that is unique. Instead of being round, the stem has two raised lines, making it appear pressed flat. The plant's tiny black seeds are carried in three-celled capsules. The erect plant smells like turpentine or balsam.

Hypericum's newborn reputation as the "People's Prozac" is a far cry from the way farmers have recently been thinking about the plant. In the western United States, parts of Australia, and South Africa, St. John's wort has been regarded as an invasive weed that needs to be vanquished forever from rangelands. It has been the bane of cowboys because it competes with native plants and threatens grazing livestock with potentially toxic sensitivity to the sun.

This tall, rangy weed carries the active compound hypericin in its narrow, lanced leaves. It's the hypericin that's responsible for the reddish stain on your skin if you rub the foliage between your fingers. Hypericin has a peculiar odor and a bitter, astringent taste. It's also most probably the source of most of the plant's healing benefits.

Still, there are more than 50 other active constituents in this plant in addition to hypericin, including pseudohypericin, flavonoids, tannins, and procyanidins. So far, scientists believe that the tannins are responsible for the astringent effect for wound healing. However, tannin and any one of these 50 compounds also might hold healing secrets we can as yet only dream about. Now vaunted as an herbal wonder drug, hypericum is no longer burned to clear evil spirits from the air. Today, it is suggested for treatments of diseases ranging from depression to AIDS, nervous system disorders, and herpes.

CHAPTER 3

Can St. John's Wort Help You?

Historically, we in the United States favor science over sleight of hand, and prescription medications over herbs. Yet the results of studies into St. John's wort involves more than hearsay and health food store hype. St. John's wort is one of the most thoroughly researched herbal medicines you can find—more than 5,000 patients have participated in European drug-monitoring studies—more than 2,000 of these in double-blind studies. Most herbs are not enthusiastically recommended by physicians because of the lack of supporting research in well-known journals to support the use of herbs. With St. John's wort, the research is encouraging.

The conclusion, reached by a variety of scientists around the world and recently published in influential journals in the United States, is that St. John's wort is more effective than a placebo in treating mild or moderate depression, and just as good (at least for a short period of time) as many standard antidepressants. Better yet, St. John's wort has far fewer side effects than antidepressant drugs—in some cases, fewer side effects than the placebo.

Still, just because we are beginning to understand more about St. John's wort doesn't mean there isn't more to know. Research to this point—although encouraging—still leaves some unanswered questions about exactly how St. John's wort works, explained Wayne Jonas, M.D., director of the U.S. Office of Alternative Medicine (OAM). Despite the number of studies, none have looked at long-term use, and published studies have used several different doses for people with differing levels of depression. We still need to know:

- How precisely does St. John's wort improve depression?
- What happens if people take St. John's wort for longer periods of time?
- Are there really no side effects, or haven't we figured out what they are yet?
- Can St. John's wort be used with severe depression?

STUDIES

First U.S. Study

Long-term studies are desperately needed, since studies that were conducted over a longer period of time (6 weeks) usually show more significant effects. To answer some of these questions, the United States in October 1997 launched the first-ever national clinical trial of St. John's wort for patients with moderate depression. The 3-year study is sponsored by the National Institute of Mental Health (NIMH), the National Institutes of Health's Office of Alternative Medicine, and the Office of Dietary Supplements.

In the study, scientists will randomly assign 336 patients diagnosed with moderate depression to 1 of 3 treatments for an 8-week trial. One third of the patients will receive a dose of St. John's wort, another third will get a placebo, and the final third will take a kind of antidepressant called a selective serotonin reuptake inhibitor (SSRI). Prozac and Paxil are two types of commonly prescribed SSRIs that have never before been compared to St. John's wort. These drugs—the newest, most modern drug treatment available for people with depression—are believed to act in the brain in very similar ways to St. John's wort.

The study will provide answers about whether St. John's wort really works for clinical depression, according to NIMH director Steven Hyman, M.D. "The study will be the first rigorous clinical trial of the herb that will be large enough and long enough to fully assess whether it produces a therapeutic effect," he says.

Scientists will also be assessing whether a longer course of treatment with the plant causes more serious side effects. While there are certainly long-term users in Germany, none of whom have reported adverse effects, only a long-term controlled clinical study can satisfy scientists that there are no risks with St. John's wort.

The U.S. study will use a standardized preparation containing a 900-mg daily dose of hypericin, the active ingredient in St. John's wort. Those who respond to the herb will be followed for another 18 weeks to determine whether patients taking St. John's wort have fewer relapses than patients given a placebo. Patient enrollment is to begin in spring 1998.

European Studies

In Europe, St. John's wort burst into worldwide medical prominence with the publication of an overview of 23 well-designed clinical studies of 1,757 patients comparing a plant extract (hypericin) with placebos or antidepressants. The overview, published in August 1996 in the *British Medical Journal,* concluded that the extract is "more effective than placebo for the treatment of mild to moderately severe depressive disorder." The study described the analysis by researchers at Ludwig-Maximilian University in Munich, who concluded that the herb was useful in cases of mild to moderate depression, since it had clearly done better than the placebo with very few side effects.

However, the reviewers refused to draw any conclusions about the future usefulness of the plant, because they believed the studies had involved too few patients. They emphasized that many issues about the use of the plant remained unclarified. It isn't known whether the extracts are as effective as traditional drugs for depression, they said, or whether the extracts are more effective for certain types of depression—or even whether they have fewer side effects.

Most of these European studies had randomly assigned depressed patients to one of two groups—one treated with St. John's wort extracts and the other treated with either a placebo or traditional antidepressant medication. The antidepressants used in these trials were amitriptyline (Elavil), desipramine (Norpramin), imipramine (Tofranil), and maprotiline (Ludiomil). Clinicians analyzed patients at the start and finish of the study using widely accepted methods of assessing depressive symptoms, usually the Hamilton Depression Rating Scale and the Clinical Global Impression Scale.

"Current evidence is inadequate to establish whether hypericum is as effective as other antidepressants," they wrote in the *British Medical Journal*. "Additional trials should be conducted to compare hypericum with other antidepressants in well-defined groups of patients." The scientists also recommended that the herb's long-term effects should be evaluated as well as the effectiveness of different preparations and dosages.

The research team who did the analysis for the *British Medical Journal*, which included scientists from Munich and San Antonio, called for more exacting studies that would compare the extract with newer antidepressants, such as Prozac. They also pointed out that the studies they reviewed involved relatively small numbers of patients, and that the diagnosis of depression varied from one study to another, without always adhering to the stringent criteria used in the United States. Moreover, the St. John's wort preparations differed from study to study, including liquid extracts, capsules, or tablets made from ground-up plants. So also were there variations in the medication's potency and dosage. Finally, none of the studies lasted longer than 8 weeks, and while few short-term side effects were found, the team cautioned that possible long-term problems with St. John's wort might have gone undiscovered.

But the results were deemed encouraging, showing that the plant was "significantly superior to placebo." Side effects, such as upset stomach, happened in less than 20 percent of participants, compared to more than half on the standard antidepressants. In a separate comment in the British journal, Netherlands clinicians Peter de Smet and Willen Nolen agreed that the data are promising, but are not yet strong enough to consider St. John's wort an effective antidepressant preparation. In addition to the need to standardize doses and conduct longer studies, the Dutch scientists call for investigations into how well hypericin works in treating severely depressed patients. They also recommend long-term studies to assess the risk of relapse and late emergence of side effects.

Since that review, other studies have been published showing the herb appears to work as well as a class of conventional antidepressants known as tricyclics (including imipramine, the "gold standard" antidepressant against which other antidepressants are often compared). Another study from Europe, which compared St. John's wort with imipramine, included 135 depressed patients at 20 different health centers. After 6 weeks of treatment, St. John's wort proved to be just as effective as the drug, but had fewer side effects. The same thing happened when the plant was compared to another antidepressant, maprotiline.

The *Journal of Geriatric Psychiatry and Neurology* devoted an entire issue, including 17 research papers, to "hypericum, a novel antidepressant." In one study that tracked the plant's effects on 3,250 patients with mild and moderate depression, 80 percent either felt better or were completely symptom free after 4 weeks.

In 1994, a randomized placebo-controlled double-blind study by a psychiatrist, an internist, and a general practitioner in Austria evaluated the effect of St. John's wort on 105 outpatients with mild to moderate depression. The study involved doses of 300 mg of either St. John's wort extract (standardized to 0.9 mg hypericin) or a placebo, three times daily for 4 weeks. Of these, 67 percent of those taking St. John's wort showed improvement compared to only 28 percent of those on the placebo. Those taking the extract felt less sad, hopeless, helpless, and fearful, they slept better, and their reported side effects were minor.

The report, and European studies in general, revealed that 50 to 80 percent of depressed patients experience a significant improvement in their depressive symptoms when they take St. John's wort. Eight other studies directly compared hypericum with antidepressants, all of which showed that the plant extract may work as well as some other prescription antidepressants in treating mild-to-moderate depression in most patients. The studies also found that hypericum had significantly fewer side effects, and that these were milder than those caused by prescription drugs.

The high rate of successful treatment, together with the minimal side effects, low cost, and availability, make hypericum an excellent choice to begin treatment for mild depression. Indeed, millions of Europeans have already done so, using hypericum daily to treat chronic depression. Hypericum also has proved effective in treating secondary symptoms of depression, such as headache, sweating, heart palpitations, anxiety, and insomnia.

At least 16 randomized, double-blind studies have found hypericum extract much more effective than a placebo. In a summary of these placebo studies, there were actually more patients who dropped out because of side effects from the "dummy" pills than with St. John's wort. This illustrates how hard it can be to tell whether physical complaints during treatment are true side effects or are caused by the depression itself. Reports of side effects also may be related to suggestions and expectations for treatment among patients in the placebo group.

In addition, there are at least eight randomized double-blind studies that compare hypericum and antidepressants, including imipramine, amitriptyline, diazepam, maprotiline, and desipramine. In general, the studies found that St. John's wort worked as well as any of the above antidepressants. In one study, however, researchers found the plant worked better than imipramine when given in a moderate dose to treat severe depression. This contradicts studies by others researchers, who only recommend St. John's wort for mild to moderate depression. More research is needed, experts say, to find out whether St. John's wort will work with severe depression.

Problems with the European studies

Still, researchers are not totally convinced that St. John's wort is the wonder drug of the new millennium, for the following reasons:

- *Symptoms.* All but one of the European studies involved only patients with mild or moderate depression, not any with a severe case. Some studies even included patients who were barely depressed at all.
- *Long-term use.* Because none of the studies has lasted longer than 6 weeks, no one knows whether the herb continues to be effective over months or years—or whether unpleasant side effects appear after long use. Animal studies suggest that high doses lead to sun sensitivity; it's possible that long-term medication may be phototoxic in humans as well.
- *Poor comparisons.* St. John's wort was tested against tricyclic antidepressants (an older class of drugs) instead of the newer SSRIs (including Prozac).
- *Improper doses.* Most of the studies compared St. John's wort with lower-than-normal doses of standard antidepressants.

St. John's wort in Germany

The results of all these studies have not surprised the Germans, a people who have never lost their connection to herbal medicine. Many traditional herbal remedies are accepted in Germany as medicines, and German manufacturers are allowed to describe the herb's use in fighting depression and anxiety on their packaging. Moreover, German health insurance must pay for the herb just as they reimburse for conventional drugs.

St. John's wort was first introduced as high-strength 300-mg extract pills in Berlin in 1992 by the Licht Wer Pharma company. Since then, sales of hypericum products have jumped to about $71 million a year, capturing 27.3 percent of the antidepressant market in Germany.

The Lichtwer company played a big role in the herb's popularity in Germany, first by offering the high-dose extract (a big improvement over oils and teas), and then by aggressively commissioning a series of respected studies of the herb at independent universities and labs.

As word spread of the little plant's big success, more and more Americans began flocking to their natural food stores in search of this natural antidepressant. An antidepressant without side effects? A cheaper, milder version of Prozac? The trickle of interest soon became a flood. An increasing number of holistic physicians—and holistic veterinarians—began using it as well. Vets use the drug to treat separation anxiety and aggression disorders in dogs and cats.

Before the first-ever U.S. study began this year, research into St. John's wort had been completed in Germany and other European countries. Since the plant is marketed as a dietary supplement in this country, the Food and Drug Administration has no jurisdiction in approving or disapproving it, and no proof is required of its safety or usefulness, as is required for prescription antidepressants. However, because it is marketed as a dietary supplement, its label may not claim that it has a specific effect in easing depression.

HYPERICUM—HOW IT WORKS

The studies seem to show *that* St. John's wort works. The problem is, no one has quite figured out exactly *how* it works.

We know the plant does not work like a tranquilizer, inducing drowsiness or euphoria. Instead, when used over long term it seems to help patients regain their overall mental balance, normalizing moods and mental attitude. German scientists have isolated compounds that seem to produce most of the herb's effects: the reddish pigment hypericin, pseudohypericin, plus xanthones and flavonoids—but how they manage to elevate mood is not known. In addition to hypericin and pseudohypericin, other substances—such as protein, fat, tannin, vitamins A and C, carotenoids, rutin, and pectin—support these activities.

Scientists suspect the active compounds in the plant work in several different ways at once. Containing more than 10 different groups of active ingredients, St. John's wort apparently acts not just on the brain, but improves the immune system at the same time, easing other symptoms associated with depression.

Most experts accept that depression is caused by a disruption in the levels of two brain chemicals—serotonin and norepinephrine. In the brain, these chemicals serve as neurotransmitters that carry nerve impulses regulating emotion and mood. Low levels of serotonin have been associated with depression for a long time; drugs like Prozac allow more serotonin to pass between cells. Hypericin and other components (particularly flavonoids) have been shown to interfere with the breakdown or reabsorption of several neurotransmitters, including serotonin. As a result, there is an increase in the level of these transmitters within the brain that helps maintain normal mood and emotional stability.

Therefore, St. John's wort seems to act on the same brain chemical system as Prozac—serotonin—and thus affect the brain much like Prozac does, by prolonging the activity of serotonin. Because drugs like Prozac are selective serotonin reuptake inhibitors (SSRIs), scientists suspect that St. John's wort might be a kind of natural SSRI. Oddly enough, the Prozac-like way that St. John's wort works in the brain doesn't seem to be the only way it alleviates depression. Rat studies also show that St. John's wort affects two other brain chemicals that are also associated with depression—dopamine and norepinephrine. The plant extract extends their action, not by stimulating their release but by preventing their reabsorption by nearby nerve fibers.

No other known antidepressant alters the levels of all three neurotransmitters at once. That fact, plus the observation that the herb has a milder tendency to bind with serotonin, may help explain why St. John's wort causes fewer side effects than other antidepressants.

But while hypericin and pseudohypericin are believed to be the active ingredients, they don't seem to be able to cross the blood-brain barrier. Some scientists think that the chemicals may act on immune cells in the rest of the body, and that these immune cells may secrete chemicals that *do* cross the blood-brain barrier—where they have to go if they are going to affect the brain.

Furthermore, a study in the 1980s suggested that some active ingredients of St. John's wort seem to decrease the action of an enzyme found in the brain called monoamine oxidase (MAO). This enzyme breaks down serotonin and other chemicals like it. If you take a drug that interferes with the action of this enzyme, you would raise the levels of serotonin—improving mood. This is exactly what another type of antidepressant drug does—the monoamine oxidase inhibitor, or MAOI (brand names Nardil or Parnate). Some scientists suspect that St. John's wort helps alleviate depression because it serves as a sort of MAOI, inhibiting the production of the monoamine oxi-dase enzyme.

While many experts still believe St. John's wort is a type of MAOI, and describe it as such, more recent studies suggest that its MAOI effect is very mild and not strong enough to account for its ability to alleviate depression. In normal doses of St. John's wort, the SSRI effect is much more prominent.

It is probably just as well, since MAOIs are among the riskiest of antidepressant drugs, with a wide range of serious side effects. They can cause the deadly "MAOI effect," in which a person's blood pres-sure can shoot up if combined with certain foods, including wine, aged cheese, liver, and smoked or pickled food. Because St. John's wort has only very slight MAOI effects, it is likely that the need to restrict your diet is not necessary. There have never been any reports of MAOI effects, although many articles still caution against combin-ing these foods with St. John's wort.

Still others suspect that the active ingredients in St. John's wort somehow lower circulating levels of the stress hormone cortisol, or that it acts on certain other receptors for a neurotransmitter substance called GABA.

In yet another intriguing discovery, scientists have found out one more thing about St. John's wort and its primary compound: Hyper-icin is capable of increasing theta waves in the brain. Theta waves normally occur during sleep, and have been associated with deep meditative states, serene pleasure, and heightened creative activity. Because of this action on theta waves, some experts think St. John's wort may be able to improve perception and clarify thinking pro-cesses.

Much Remains Unknown

While the results from a variety of studies are intriguing, there is still a lot more that scientists need to know. There are no well-established doses of the herbal extract. In the European studies, doses of the hypericin compound ranged from 0.48 to 2.7 mg. The flavonoids and xanthones weren't measured at all. Doctors caution against wildly embracing St. John's wort in the way that many people leapt on the Prozac bandwagon. While many people like the idea of a natural herb, St. John's wort is not always effective. But it is one treatment that is successful with some people in some situations.

CHAPTER 4

Where to Buy St. John's Wort

When your doctor prescribes an antidepressant, you know that when you go to the drugstore you'll be coming home with a bottle of pills containing exactly the ingredients the doctor has ordered. There isn't much choice about the form of that drug, where you buy it, or what it contains.

When it comes to St. John's wort, you're facing a completely different situation. Hypericum is sold in a variety of different formulations—extracts, tinctures, tablets, and capsules. You can order it through the mail, from a natural food store, or from a health food store.

REGULATION

Remember that the U.S. Food and Drug Administration (FDA) does not regulate St. John's wort, which is sold not as a medication but as a food supplement. Products that you find on your health food store shelves have not been checked by any governmental agency for either contents or potency. The bottle, therefore, may or may not contain what the label says it does. There are no guarantees that pills purchased in health food stores contain the dosage the label claims—or that they even contain the active ingredient at all. Manufacturers can legally call a product "hypericum" or St. John's wort, even if it contains only an infinitesimal quantity of the herb. Experts note that many products in health food stores contain overly diluted concentrations that render the plant impotent.

The best dosage—based on the majority of research studies—is 300 mg of hypericum extract, containing 0.3 percent of the active ingredient (hypericin), taken three times a day. Allow at least 3 weeks before you expect to see improvement. However, since there are so many preparations of St. John's wort, you should do the math for whatever brand you buy.

The FDA, a division of the department of Health and Human Services, is the federal agency that administers and enforces the federal Food, Drug, and Cosmetic Act of 1938, which provides the basis for the regulation of much of the testing, manufacture, distribution, and sale of food, drugs, cosmetics, and medical devices that are sold to the public. The FDA's job is to protect consumers by preventing unsupported or insubstantial information on food and dietary supplement labeling.

Unlike European countries, the United States has done very little research on whole plants as medicinal substances. In the United States, a plant cannot be patented. American drug companies screen plants for biological activity, and isolate active compounds. If the active compounds seem to be powerful enough, the drug companies start the process for a new drug application for FDA approval. This is a costly and time-consuming process, and there usually isn't much financial incentive for a drug company to start this process.

To make sure the American public has over-the-counter access to dietary supplements (including vitamins, minerals, amino acids, herbs, and botanicals), Congress passed the Dietary Supplement Health and Education Act of 1994. The act specifically forbids the FDA from regulating any dietary supplement as a drug, unless the FDA finds the product isn't safe.

Still, there isn't any formal way to check health claims for herbs without going through a "new drug application" process—a huge commitment beyond the scope of most herb companies. At present, all that is required on the labeling for dietary supplements is that the information must be truthful, nonmisleading, scientifically backed "statements of nutritional support." The labels can include "structure and function claims" to describe how a supplement alters the structure or function of the body.

WHERE TO BUY ST. JOHN'S WORT

St. John's wort is currently available as an elixir (dissolved in grain alcohol) and in capsule form in U.S. health food stores across the country. Companies that follow European manufacturing standards use the word *standardized* on the label, together with a list of the amount of herb and the percentage of hypericin. A 300-mg capsule of 0.3 percent hypericin is an amount about equal to the doses used in the European studies. It's also available dried and in concentrated drops and tinctures.

In the United States, St. John's wort is usually harvested in July and August. If more herb is needed, it won't be necessary to wait another year, since the same plant species is common in Australia. You should be able to find the plant in any health food store, sold either as "St. John's wort" or by its botanical name, "hypericum." Remember that the active ingredient is "hypericin," which also may appear on the label. St. John's wort is available through naturopaths, herbalists, and other natural healers, or you can get your own through mail order (see Appendix A). You'll also find an extensive list of suppliers online through hypericum Web sites (see Appendix F).

Of course, in Germany, where hypericum is a registered medicine, you'd be able to buy the herb via prescription from your family doctor. In Germany, St. John's wort is sold as Jarsin, Kari, Psychotonin, Neuroplant, and others.

FORMS OF ST. JOHN'S WORT

Extracts

Many companies simply grind up the plant, process it into capsules, and call it "hypericum" or St. John's wort. But that's not the way the research-grade hypericum used in most medical studies is produced. Eventually, research may show that this method of producing St. John's wort is perfectly acceptable, but at the moment alcohol extraction is the only method of preparation that has been medically proven to be successful in treating depression.

An extract is made by dissolving the crushed flowering and/or leafy portions of the *Hypericum perforatum* plant in alcohol or glycerin, allowing the oily active ingredients to dissolve into the liquid. When the alcohol evaporates, the extract remains and the inactive residue is strained out. The extract is then tested and adjusted, so that the strength of each batch is the same. There isn't any alcohol left over in the final product—the alcohol is simply used to extract the medically useful chemicals from the plant.

This is why drinking tea made from St. John's wort may not be nearly as effective. No studies have been done comparing "water-extracted" St. John's wort with alcohol extractions of the plant.

The extract formula used in the medical studies and widely sold in Britain is marketed under the brand names Jarsin or Jarsin 300—products which are not currently available in this country under those names. However, this formula is available under a variety of other brand names (see Appendix B), sold both in retail stores and through the mail.

Liquid extracts are usually sold in small brown glass bottles with a screw-on medicine dropper top. The dark glass protects the extract from deteriorating as a result of exposure to light. It's a good idea to store your liquid extract in the refrigerator to protect against heat-related deterioration. Read the labels to make sure the herbs were harvested in the wild, away from roadsides and areas that might have been sprayed with herbicides. Commercial extracts are standardized to contain a certain percentage of hypericin. For correct dosage, follow the directions on the bottle.

Remember that extracts come from different parts of the plants. If you compare brands, you'll see that some are prepared from the buds of St. John's wort, while others are made from the unopened flowering tops of the plant. If the label doesn't go into details, this suggests that the extract was probably prepared with the buds and leaves—it's cheaper that way for the producer.

Most herbalists will tell you that when you're shopping for St. John's wort, you should choose extracts made from the buds. Because the buds contain the highest proportion of the active ingredients, an extract made from buds is probably more potent. This doesn't mean that other brands or methods are worthless. They all contain active ingredients, and some herbalists swear that it's better to use a product made from the entire St. John's wort plant—buds, stems, leaves, roots, and all—since only by using the whole plant can you be sure of getting all of the active components. These herbalists will tell you that since no one yet knows exactly which constituents of the plant are responsible for which healing properties, it makes sense to use the whole herb as a way of increasing your chances of getting the most potent compounds.

There have been no studies that looked at whether buds or leaves have a stronger effect against depression or any other health problem.

Tinctures

Tinctures are alcohol-based extracts, and usually contain more alcohol than extracts—sometimes up to 70 or 80 percent alcohol, depending on the manufacturer. A tincture, like an extract, offers the advantage of high concentration in low weight and space. Several brands are available in natural food stores.

Capsules and Tablets

Capsules and tablets are one of the fastest growing markets in herbal medicine—they're convenient and neat, and you don't have to taste the herb when you take them. Tablets are made by harvesting the flowers and leaves, and then drying and processing them into a powdered extract. The powder is shaped into a pill, coated with sugar, dried, and packaged. Some brands of tablets are made from standardized extracts, but many are not, so different brands may well have different strengths. The directions on each label therefore must be closely followed.

While St. John's wort capsules and tablets are available at most natural food stores, herbalists generally prefer extracts. The problem with capsules and tablets, or raw dried herbs, is that it's hard to tell how potent they are because exposure to light and air may break down the active ingredients.

In some of the depression studies, scientists used extract capsules of 900 mg daily. Each dose, however, was standardized to ensure that exactly the same amount of hypericin (1 mg) was given in each dose.

Oils

Good quality oils are available at natural food stores. Look for bottles with a rich, red color, signifying that the compound was made when the flowers were freshest.

The oil will keep for up to 2 years if stored in a dark place.

Teas

You can buy herbal tea loose, but it's not usually recommended to get your St. John's wort with this method—it's just not strong enough.

Combination Herbs

Many herbs are sold in combination products, such as the "women's tonics" that include St. John's wort together with a host of other herbs. Many herbalists do not recommend this shotgun approach, since it can be difficult to tell how you will respond to this compound. In addition, if you have an allergic reaction or unpleasant side effects, it may be impossible to figure out which herb in the product was responsible.

AT THE STORE

Buying organic?

When choosing your St. John's wort, you might as well select an organic product, since organically grown herbs tend to be tougher, with higher concentrations of active ingredients. Look for the organic certification on the label; this means that the grower has passed strict regular inspections that guarantee the product is not covered in pesticides.

If the label mentions that the herb has been "wildcrafted," this indicates it was harvested from wild-growing plants, not those that have been cultivated. This could be important, since many herbalists believe that the plant grows best and healthiest when not overly cultivated, but allowed to grow free—like the weed it really is.

Decoding the Label

One of the problems with buying St. John's wort at a health food store is that there's such a variety of products from which to choose. The label will usually give a range of suggested doses; you should choose the average, middle dose to begin with and see how you do on that. If the label recommends you take between 20 and 40 drops, opt for 30 and then evaluate your response. The very young or the very old, however, should lean toward the lowest possible dose and then work upward if that is not satisfactory.

Most labels will also contain information about how strong the extract is—with wording such as "Fresh herb strength 1:1," which means how much of the ground fresh herb was added to how much of the alcohol (or glycerin).

Note that not every U.S. manufacturer standardizes their extracts or tablets, so the amount of active ingredients may vary from one batch to the next. While this may seem alarming, St. John's wort is so nontoxic that there is much less risk in this irregularity. The herb extracts are far more standardized in Europe.

COST

At between $8 and $10 for a month's supply, St. John's wort is significantly cheaper than most antidepressant drugs (especially the newer medicines that are not available as generic). For example, Prozac and similar SSRIs cost about $70 to $80 a month at a discount pharmacy.

CHAPTER 5

How to Use St. John's Wort

In Germany, hypericin is used to treat nearly half of all cases of depression, anxiety, and sleep disorders. But in order to get the best from this preparation, you'll have to make some decisions: Capsule or tablet, tincture or extract? Standardized? Mixed with other ingredients, or just the active ingredient?

In the case of St. John's wort, studies have been very clear: it *does* matter what preparation of the plant you take if you want to get the biggest bang for your buck. Most herbalists prefer St. John's wort—or its active compound, hypericin—taken as an alcohol extract.

HOW TO TAKE ST. JOHN'S WORT

Most of the studies that have looked at St. John's wort have concluded that the best dosage is 300 mg of hypericum extract (0.3 percent hypericin) three times a day. Most people do well on a schedule of extract taken in the morning upon arising—say, 7 a.m. The next dose would then be taken at 10 a.m. and the final dose at 1 p.m. (that is, 3 hours apart). Others prefer taking two doses at breakfast, and a third at lunch.

If you take the alcohol extract, you can divide three-quarters of a teaspoon into two or three doses per day. If you choose a capsule instead, look for brands containing 300 mg of raw herb, standardized to contain 0.3 percent hypericin. Take one capsule three times a day—less if you are over age 65.

Patients who think that St. John's wort helps them sleep can spread out their doses, reserving the final amount to be taken at dinner or bedtime.

Since the side effects of St. John's wort are rare even in significantly higher doses, you could take four 250-mg capsules a day, if the only herb you can find occurs in 250-mg capsules.

If you are between ages 12 and 45, are basically healthy, and take the herb for a short time, no risks are expected.

After 6 weeks, you should evaluate how you're doing on the 900-mg-a-day schedule. (It may take this long to notice an effect, just as it can take months to notice the effects of antidepressants.) Studies indicate that it can take hypericum longer to reach its full effectiveness than prescription antidepressants.

Take with Meals

You should take St. John's wort on a full stomach to avoid the potential of nausea and stomach upset. If you take any product on an empty stomach, your stomach lining can be irritated by the intense concentration of chemicals.

St. John's wort is not one of the medications that is inactivated in the presence of food—so wait until mealtime to take your herb. It's a good way to remember when to take your next dose, anyway.

Storage

Keep St. John's wort cool and dry, but don't freeze it. Store safely away from children. At present, no "safe" dose has been established. It is rated "slightly dangerous" in children, those over age 55, and those who take larger-than-appropriate amounts for long periods of time.

GAUGING YOUR RESPONSE TO ST. JOHN'S WORT

How Soon You'll Respond

Don't take this herb one night and expect to have a response by the next morning. Like all antidepressants, St. John's wort must be taken for several weeks before a response is noted—usually up to a month. Still, many consumers notice some response by day 10. Remember that this herb is not a synthetic manufactured drug—it's gentle, and it's mild. Results will probably be very slight at first, but will strengthen as time goes on.

Length of Treatment

One of the toughest questions to answer about any antidepressant is how long to take it. In general, doctors advise patients not to take prescription antidepressant drugs longer than 6 months to a year, although some people need to continue medication for a year or more.

Since no long-term studies have been conducted on hypericum, experts don't recommend that people take it for more than a year. While it is true that the plant has been prescribed by herbalists for thousands of years with no reported deaths, it's probably prudent to avoid long-term use until more research has been done.

When you decide to stop taking St. John's wort, you should do so gradually, cutting down the dose slowly over about a month. (However, if you've decided to stop taking hypericum because of side effects, you can stop immediately, if you must.)

IF YOU DON'T RESPOND

If you feel that you have not responded to St. John's wort, then you should consult with your doctor and discuss taking a prescription antidepressant instead. Not everyone responds to the first traditional antidepressant they take, and not everyone responds to St. John's wort, either.

Depression *can* be treated successfully, and should be treated promptly. Even though prescription antidepressants may cost more and have more side effects, if St. John's wort doesn't work and your doctor believes prescription antidepressants are necessary, you shouldn't hesitate to try them.

There are many different antidepressants available. If one isn't successful, or if the side effects are a problem, there are many others from which to choose. You need to work with your doctor to find the right prescription for you.

For this reason, it's very important not to decide after only a week or two that St. John's wort isn't helping your depression—it almost always takes at least a month for the full effect of hypericum to be felt.

Side Effects

Of course, if you do experience severe unpleasant side effects, you should consult your health care provider immediately. All symptoms should stop within a few days after the last dose is taken. It is true, however, that many of the side effects (especially the milder ones) disappear after your body becomes adjusted to the herb. It may help if you decrease your dosage slightly until your body gets accustomed to St. John's wort. **If the side effects of your depression become worse, or you begin having suicidal thoughts, see your doctor immediately.** (See Chapter 6 for more information.)

PRECAUTIONS ABOUT ST. JOHN'S WORT

Experts suggest pregnant or breastfeeding women should avoid this herb. Anyone who is taking St. John's wort should avoid the following:

- alcoholic beverages
- medications such as narcotics, amphetamines, and over-the-counter cold and flu remedies
- prescription antidepressants
- excessive exposure to sunlight

The Young

While most people think of depression as an adults' disease, in fact at least 2 percent of children and 5 percent of teenagers suffer from clinical depression. Many antidepressants have not been studied in children under age 12, and scientists aren't sure what the risks would be. It's a concern of experts who must treat depression in the young, whose still-developing nervous system may be affected by these drugs.

Experts recommend that small children take just 300 mg total a day, while larger children can take 600 mg a day. Teenagers can handle an adult dose. The fact that St. John's wort appears to have very few side effects makes it a much more attractive choice in treating young people. Experts point out that treating any infant or child under age 2 with any herbal preparation—including St. John's wort—can be hazardous.

The Elderly

People over age 65 and those who are chronically or severely ill are more likely than the rest of us to suffer from depression. Unfortunately, the same people are more susceptible to the side effects of traditional antidepressants. In other cases, conventional antidepressants may interact unpleasantly with other medications the elderly are already taking.

For these reasons, St. John's wort may be a particular benefit, since the rare side effects are not serious in most cases. However, caution must be used when taking St. John's wort, since the elderly in general tend to become more sensitive to medications of all types with age.

For this reason, consumers over age 65 should use a smaller dose of St. John's wort, no matter whether you're using an extract, capsule, tablet, or dried herb. Read the label carefully, and take the lowest recommended dose for about a month before evaluating your response. Increase the dose only if you haven't responded by then.

To be safe, herbalists recommend that if the bottle gives just one standard dose, you should halve that dose. If the label directs you to take 20 drops twice a day, you should take 10 drops twice a day for a month, then see how you're feeling.

CHAPTER 6

Side Effects

St. John's wort is one of our very oldest medicinal herbs, and it has amassed an excellent safety record through the centuries. In Germany during 1994 alone, there were 66 million doses taken without any reports of a single serious drug interaction, or even toxicity after accidental overdose.

Other than a potential harmful interaction with other antidepressants (which has never happened, but that scientists are worried about), there are few side effects with St. John's wort. Those that do appear are fairly rare. In fact, herbal experts believe that the plant is safer than aspirin. Between 500 and 1,000 people die every year as a result of reactions to aspirin (usually internal bleeding). Hypericum, on the other hand, has not been responsible for a single recorded death in the 2,400 years of recorded medical history. That's an impressive record.

Of course, no substance can be completely safe. Even table salt is toxic in large doses. When reading about side effects, it may help to compare one substance with another. You may have a serious reaction if you overdose on aspirin, for example, but it's still a safer drug than morphine.

In trying to assess whether a substance's side effects are serious, it may also help to look at the illness it is trying to cure. Many of the side effects of chemotherapy, for example, are devastating, but compared to the disease which they are trying to suppress—cancer—many patients are willing to accept constant nausea and hair loss for a chance to live longer.

In fact, one of the reasons scientists are so interested in hypericum is that side effects are so rare, and those that do occur are nontoxic. In one study of 3,250 patients, only 2.4 percent experienced any side effects. Of these, 0.6 percent were gastrointestinal, 0.5 percent had an allergic reaction, 0.4 percent got tired, and 0.3 percent felt restless. Those side effects that did appear with hypericum faded away when the plant was stopped. St. John's wort caused no permanent damage.

Slightly more side effects were noted in a review of six hypericum studies, as reported in the *British Medical Journal*. In this review, 10.8 percent of people taking St. John's wort reported side effects (similar to the complaints mentioned above), compared to 35.9 percent who reported side effects from antidepressants.

Remember, too, that some of the "side effects" people report while using a substance may be coincidental, having nothing to do with the medication. In fact, in 15 studies of 1,008 people, the rate of side effects in the placebo groups—that is, the groups taking "dummy pills" containing no active ingredients—was a bit higher than the rate of side effects reported with the hypericum group. The dropout rate in the placebo group was higher, too. A total of 4 percent of patients receiving extract dropped out of the trial because of side effects; 7.7 percent of those receiving standard antidepressants dropped out due to side effects.

It's also important to keep in mind that the side effects that were reported with St. John's wort are mild ones. The side effects that occur with antidepressants are much more bothersome, including reduced sexual drive or dysfunction, adverse interaction with alcohol or other drugs, dry mouth, and headache. None of these side effects occurred with St. John's wort.

Keep in mind the dangers of the alternative: The side effects of depression can be extreme. About 70 percent of all suicides (21,000 deaths) are the direct result of an untreated depression, and for every suicide, there are 10 other unsuccessful attempts and another 100 people who are seriously thinking about it. Untreated depression is also the main cause of alcoholism, drug abuse, eating disorders, and other addictions, and is linked to divorce, abuse, absenteeism, and lost jobs.

When studies compare side effects of St. John's wort with those of standard antidepressants, participants rate the side effects of the plant as far less intense than those of antidepressant drugs. This means that even when a side effect does appear, it is usually much milder than a side effect that occurs from taking an antidepressant drug.

The most commonly reported side effects associated with hypericum include fatigue, skin rash/itching, and stomach problems. If you experience any of these symptoms and they seem fairly mild, you may choose to continue taking St. John's wort. Sometimes, as your body gets used to the plant, these side effects fade away.

If you do experience any side effects, you should at least tell your doctor right away. There is one interaction that is of great concern to experts, and that is the potential interaction between St. John's wort and antidepressants, which we'll discuss next.

ANTIDEPRESSANT INTERACTION

The most serious problem that can occur with St. John's wort is a potential one—it's something that scientists worry about, but that to anyone's knowledge has not yet happened—and that is the possible interaction with other antidepressants. Just as it can be very dangerous to switch from certain types of antidepressants to certain other kinds, it can be dangerous to switch from an antidepressant to St. John's wort, or vice versa. For the same reason, it could be dangerous to take the plant and an antidepressant at the same time.

What You Can Do

There is almost no research that has been done on the safety of these antidepressants and St. John's wort—just anecdotal evidence. Doctors are particularly concerned with the selective serotonin reuptake inhibitors (SSRIs, such as Prozac) or the older antidepressant monoamine oxidase inhibitors (MAOIs).

Here are the guidelines:

1. *Do not* abruptly stop taking prescription antidepressants without your doctor's knowledge and approval. The effect of suddenly going off your medication can be severe.

2. Do not take hypericum for severe depression or manic-depressive illness (bipolar disorder). There has not been enough research on the interaction between this plant and these types of depression. A "severe depression" may be clearly debilitating, include hallucinations or suicide attempts, or require hospitalization. Your doctor is the best person to determine who is and who isn't "severely" depressed.

3. **Do not take hypericum while taking monoamine oxidase inhibitors (MAOIs)** such as Nardil or Parnate. Scientists think that hypericum may mimic the effects of an antidepressant drug class known as selective serotonin reuptake inhibitors (SSRIs), like Prozac. Combining an SSRI with an MAOI can cause sudden severe high blood pressure.

4. After stopping MAOIs, you should wait *4 weeks* before taking any SSRI, either the prescription drug or hypericum. Scientists don't know for sure (research hasn't been done) if there is a serious problem between the two, but the warning has been issued because of what is known about SSRIs and MAOIs.

Unfortunately, the best way to make the change from one of the SSRIs (Prozac, Paxil, Zoloft, or Effexor) to St. John's wort isn't known, either. However, if the plant and the drug work in roughly the same way, experts suspect the best way to make the transition would be to gradually taper off one and onto the other.

Because St. John's wort takes longer to reach its full effect than do prescription antidepressants, herbalists suspect that it may make sense to gradually increase the dosage of St. John's wort *before* significantly reducing the prescription antidepressant.

It is also important to avoid taking too much SSRIs to avoid "serotonin syndrome"—a condition where the brain gets too much serotonin (the opposite of what happens in depression), causing agitation or lethargy, confusion, tremor, and muscle jerks. If you experience any of these symptoms, see your doctor immediately.

Just because you responded well to an antidepressant drug doesn't mean that you will automatically respond well to St. John's wort. Keep in mind that some people will not do as well on the plant.

DIET DRUG INTERACTIONS

Again, while there is a lack of research that has found a problem in mixing St. John's wort with diet drugs, experts believe that it is safe to assume any substance that works on serotonin levels in the brain—as St. John's wort does—may interact with other similar-acting drugs.

Taking St. John's wort with the new weight-loss drug Redux, or another popular diet drug combination, fen-phen (fenfluramine and phentermine, sold as Pondimin and Ionaminsee), might cause adverse reactions. Fen-phen raises the levels of serotonin in the brain, reducing the craving for certain foods.

PHOTOTOXICITY

One of the most common side effects in animals is related to the skin, which is why you will sometimes find St. John's wort listed as an "unsafe" drug. Animal studies using high doses of St. John's wort have noted skin inflammation after sun exposure (phototoxicity). This also has occurred outside the lab, in certain light-skinned animals (such as sheep) who died from extreme sunburn as a result of exposure after eating the plant. This is why in some areas of the west, ranchers attack St. John's wort with herbicides.

While theoretically possible in humans, such a severe skin reaction has never been documented in the doses recommended to treat depression. Even in AIDS research studies using doses of intravenous hypericum 35 times above the recommended dose for depression, only a few phototoxic effects were noted. None were fatal. In one large drug-monitoring study of 3,250 people taking St. John's wort, skin problems were noted in about 1 out of every 300 people (0.3 percent). The photosensitivity disappeared after the drug was stopped.

The photosensitizer in St. John's wort is hypericin, one of the primary active compounds of the plant responsible for giving the extract its red color.

Scientists understand that the photosensitizing effects of St. John's wort occur only when consumed in huge quantities—the Australian sheep who died as a result, for example, ate St. John's wort as their main source of food. Used in normal amounts as a medication in humans, only about 1 out of every 300 would become sensitive to sunlight as a result. This photosensitivity occurs most often in fair-haired, blue-eyed Caucasians, since these people have the least amount of natural pigment in their skin that protects against the harmful rays of the sun.

What You Can Do

It's important to understand that the photosensitizing effects of this plant are preventable. If you are normally extremely sensitive to sunlight and you choose to take St. John's wort, it's a good idea to either stay out of the sun (at least between 10 a.m. and 2 p.m.) or use plenty of sunblock and wear sunglasses and a hat when you go outdoors. Since photosensitivity is related to the amount of St. John's wort you're taking, if you have fair skin, consider reducing your dose of St. John's wort in the summer months.

Of course, dermatologists will tell you that whether or not you're taking St. John's wort, you shouldn't be spending hours in the sun without protecting your skin anyway. It's always a good idea to use a good sunscreen whenever you have to be in the sun, to cut down on your chance of melanoma (skin cancer).

Regardless of skin type, if you are taking St. John's wort you should also be careful about sun exposure if you are taking other photosensitizing drugs, such as chlorpromazine or tetracycline.

If a sunburn-like rash does develop, get out of direct sunlight as quickly as possible, and stop taking the herb. Later, you could switch to a smaller dose, but you might want to consider alternative therapy.

STOMACH PROBLEMS

The most common side effects reported by about 1 in every 200 people who take St. John's wort are nausea, appetite loss, stomach pain, and diarrhea. These symptoms are often found in people who are stressed or depressed, so they may not be related to the plant.

What You Can Do

Just in case your stomach problems are related to taking St. John's wort, here are some hints to help you deal with these side effects:

- Dilute the extract in a large glass of water to decrease its concentration in your stomach. Or mix it with a large bottle of spring water and sip it all day long—just be sure to drink all the water by the end of the day.
- Don't take St. John's wort on an empty stomach.
- Spread your total dose of the extract out over the day, as

often as five times a day (but don't take any *more* than the normal daily dose—just take it in smaller amounts). If you had been taking it three times a day, instead divide the same amount of the extract this way: with your breakfast at 7 a.m., with a snack at 10 a.m., with lunch at 1 p.m., with a snack at 4 p.m., with dinner at 7 p.m.

- Avoid substances that can irritate your stomach—dairy products, greasy food, pickled products, alcohol, caffeine, and smoking.
- Try some ginger ale—ginger is a known stomach soother. It's best to drink flat ginger ale at room temperature (cold beverages will irritate an upset stomach). Take tiny sips, especially if you have already vomited. If you can keep that down, sip a bit more.
- If you're out of ginger ale, you can try making a cup of ginger tea (with grated gingerroot). Some people even find relief by nibbling on a gingersnap.
- If you feel very nauseated, try nibbling on some plain saltine crackers.
- Don't take vitamin supplements at the same time as you take St. John's wort.
- Substitute the glycerin-based extract for the alcohol-based extract.
- Substitute a plain extract for a flavored one.
- If nothing else eases your queasy stomach, cut the dose of St. John's wort and see if that helps.

FATIGUE

Experts aren't sure why so many antidepressants cause fatigue in people who take them, but about 1 out of every 250 people who take St. John's wort will also experience this side effect. St. John's wort doesn't have a sedative effect, so herbalists don't know why fatigue may be a problem in some people.

What You Can Do

If you are feeling extra tired when you take St. John's wort, it may be linked to your depression, or to an unhealthy lifestyle. Make sure you're eating right, and getting enough exercise and plenty of rest. Cut down on your caffeine and alcohol consumption. If fatigue is really a problem and it doesn't go away in a few days, think about going off St. John's wort and see what happens. If you're still tired, the fatigue may not have had anything to do with the plant.

ANXIETY

Very rarely—in just about 1 out of every 400 people in one study— St. John's wort appeared to cause anxiety and palpitations. This side effect is often associated also with Prozac, affecting about 1 in every 11 people. Because St. John's wort and Prozac (and other similar drugs in Prozac's class) work in similar ways, it's not surprising that they can both be related to anxiety.

What You Can Do

The anxiety related to St. John's wort is very, very rare and of a mild nature. If you do experience anxiety and believe it's related to the plant, you may want to see if the anxiety passes in a day or so. Patients taking Prozac, which causes a much more severe form of anxiety, have noted that the problem does go away after a week or two.

You might try decreasing your dosage temporarily, to see if this helps your anxiety. If you feel uncomfortable, of course, you can always stop taking St. John's wort.

ALLERGIC RESPONSE

It's possible for an individual to be allergic to just about anything, so it's not surprising that a few folks may be allergic to St. John's wort. In one large drug-monitoring study, about 1 in every 500 people had an allergic response characterized by an itchy skin rash, nausea, abdominal pain, or diarrhea. Of course, some of these same symptoms may also appear with St. John's wort, and they have nothing to do with an allergic response. This is why you need to discuss any allergies with your doctor.

What You Can Do

The allergic responses discussed above are not life threatening. However, it is theoretically possible that someone can have such a severe response—called an anaphylactic response—to any drug or plant. This would cause swelling of the lips, tongue, or throat and airways (cutting off the air supply). Any such swelling or breathing problems indicate an emergency situation. Call 911 or an ambulance immediately and seek medical care.

DRY MOUTH

Dry mouth is usually more of an annoyance than anything else, but it was reported by about 6 percent of the participants in one study.

What You Can Do

If you are bothered by dry mouth, you could try the following:

- Suck on a piece of hard candy or a throat lozenge.
- Carry a bottle of spring water with you and sip often. (Most people don't drink enough water anyway.)

The problem with most antidepressants is that so many of them cause dizziness, because they interfere with the way your body controls blood pressure. If blood pressure falls, you don't get enough blood to your brain when you stand up, and you can faint. This is a particular problem among older people, who can become severely injured during a faint-induced fall.

St. John's wort causes dizziness much less often than do prescription antidepressants, but it still can occur. In one recent study, dizziness was reported in fewer than 1 out of every 650 people.

What You Can Do

If you're one of those rare people who get dizzy when you take St. John's wort, try these tips:

- If you've been sitting or lying down for a long time, stand up slowly so that your blood pressure has time to adapt to the change.
- Despite these precautions, if you feel dizzy, stop whatever you're doing and get your head lower than your heart. Put your head between your knees, for example, to allow more blood to flood into your brain. Then, taking your time, raise your head slowly. Don't stand up until you're sure the dizzy spell has passed.
- If your dizziness is really severe, you may want to stop taking St. John's wort. However, you probably run a higher risk of this same symptom with other antidepressants.
- Talk to your doctor about other options for raising your blood pressure.

OTHER SIDE EFFECTS

Some side effects are reported with St. John's wort that are so infrequent, they may be simple coincidences. These have occurred in less than 1 out of every 1,000 people, and include the following:

- weakness
- sleep problems

CHAPTER 7

Growing Your Own

St. John's wort is easy to transplant or start from seed, but before you do, you need to understand that in many parts of the country it's considered a noxious weed. If you do introduce this plant into your herb garden, watch carefully that it doesn't escape cultivation. Native to Europe, St. John's wort has naturalized throughout many parts of North America, where you can find it most often in woods and meadows, and along some roadsides. Yet the lengths to which governments and ranchers have gone to destroy this plant is tangible proof that many plants are "weeds" only because we cannot recognize their usefulness.

A final caveat: If you want to grow your own St. John's wort for medicinal purposes, it's important to understand that the best results come from buying standardized, "research-grade" versions of the plant. When you grow a plant, the amount of active compound inside the plant depends on soil type, water, sun, and nutrients. One plant may have a wildly different amount of hypericin, one of the most active medicinal ingredients in St. John's wort. Buying a standardized version of the extract means that the producer has combined many plants and then made sure each one includes exactly the same amount of active compound.

GROWING YOUR OWN

If you're sure you want to grow your own, the seeds of St. John's wort can be found at nurseries or by mail order (see Appendix C). The plants are easily started from seeds, and can be propagated by cuttings or division in spring or late fall.

The plants also can be propagated by cuttings or division in the fall. Because it grows wild, you may choose to transplant some good-sized wild plants to your own nursery beds by digging them up intact. Although it spreads by runners, St. John's wort isn't necessarily invasive, and it can be controlled by pulling out the young shoots.

Hardy to zone 5, St. John's wort tolerates average to poor soil that is either acid or alkaline, with part shade to full sun. It grows especially well in abandoned or disrupted soil, with some protection for its roots. Indeed, like many herbs, it seems to do better when not fussed over but left to survive and prosper on its own. It does prefer fairly well drained soil; if it gets too much water it won't flourish.

If you do choose to plant it from seed, remember where this herb originally comes from—it's a weed, and it does best when you treat it like a weed. If you get seeds, don't plant them in neat rows the way you would treat other herbs or vegetables. Herbalists and gardeners report that when planted this way, it seems to attract beetles that kill the plant. Don't plant in large quantities, or sow it among other plants. You can find it at all elevations, but the higher you grow it, the less oil it will yield.

Once you've planted the seeds or plants, water during droughts and provide cover on very cold nights. (Freezing will kill the plant.)

FIRST-YEAR GROWTH

The plant will only grow about 3 or 4 inches tall the first year; in winter it will die back to the earth, but will grow again in the spring. It will live this way—dying back in winter and blooming again the next year—for several years, eventually reaching 1 or 2 feet in height. If you've got a really healthy plant in just the right place, it could reach as high as 3 feet.

While many herbalists and organic farmers insist this plant is not invasive, it is considered a noxious plant by nonorganic farming standards, especially in the western states. Your neighbors may not be pleased that you're growing this particular plant. Because of this plant's effect on some grazing herds, the governments of Canada, Australia (where sheep are especially troubled by this plant), and South Africa have funded projects to develop pesticides that would wipe out St. John's wort. In the United States, the agriculture department has been trying to destroy St. John's wort for the last 50 years without success.

HARVEST TIPS

The plants usually flower during July and August, producing bright yellow flowers on a 2-foot bushy green shrub. St. John's wort is less sensitive to frost, and its flowering tops and stems can also be used to obtain red and yellow dyes.

Harvest the tops when the plants are in full bloom, usually in the morning of early to mid-July. Clip off the flowers and make a tincture or an oil infusion (see Appendix L for recipes) as soon after harvest as possible, because this plant is most potent if used for medicine when it's fresh. Otherwise, dry and store in a dark place.

If you are harvesting the leaves, these also should be picked in the morning, then dried and stored in a dark place. Old plants contain the greatest amount of the active compound (hypericin); the young plants seem to be the most toxic to livestock. The fresh leaves may be pressed for their oil and then added to olive or other vegetable oils. Preparations of St. John's wort oil will turn red with age and keep for about 2 years. Otherwise, you should dry the plant for future use.

GROWING IT INDOORS

If you're strapped for outdoor garden space, you can try growing St. John's wort indoors in wide, shallow pots. The soil should include two parts peat, two parts regular garden soil, one part compost or composted manure, and one part sand. Plant and water well; add water when the soil is dry. Make sure the pots get plenty of sun—at least 6 hours a day. If your house is facing the wrong direction for this much sun, you could invest in a grow-light.

CHAPTER 8

Other Uses for St. John's Wort

According to herbal tradition, St. John's wort is a profoundly useful medicinal plant in ways far removed from its action as an antidepressant. For thousands of years, the plant has been used to treat wounds, burns, infections, and pain. It was given as a nerve tonic and an antibacterial, an anti-inflammatory and an antiviral, long before the existence of sophisticated pharmaceutical preparations.

For those of us accustomed to one drug specifically designed for one treatment, this all-purpose medicinal plant makes many people—especially scientists—uneasy. The more illnesses a plant is said to cure, the more it reminds us of early American snake-oil salesmen and charlatans hawking useless cure-alls that did more harm than good.

Before we jump to this conclusion, however, it may help to remember that some drugs do, in fact, have more than one use. The ever-popular Prozac, for instance, was first licensed to treat depression. But it has proved to be of use for social anxiety, obsessive-compulsive disorder, bulimia, anorexia, PMS, alcoholism, nicotine withdrawal, dementia, Tourette's syndrome, exhibitionism, panic attacks—everything from itchy skin to the more severe mental illnesses such as schizophrenia or borderline personality disorder.

It shouldn't be surprising that St. John's wort may successfully treat more than one problem, given that it contains hundreds of different compounds, each with separate and unique effects. Surprisingly, some European studies of St. John's wort suggest that the plant really may be able to soothe inflammation, fight viruses and bacteria, heal wounds—and even attack HIV and cancer cells. In addition to the antidepressant-like hypericin contained in the plant, scientists have discovered dozens of other chemical compounds in St. John's wort that possess a wide range of healing properties against bacteria, fungi, and even viruses. These compounds include essential oils, flavonoids, tannins, and phytosterols.

In Germany, where all medical students must study herbal medicine as part of their medical curriculum, 40 percent of practicing physicians prescribe herbal medicines. They are aided in their practice by the German government, which publishes a series of reports to guide the herbal industry and health care providers in the use of herbs. In this report, the uses for St. John's wort include treatment of fear and nervous disorders, digestive disturbances, sharp/abrasive wounds, muscle pain, and first-degree burns.

Before beginning this discussion of the variety of ways St. John's wort has been used in the laboratory to treat other diseases, it is important to understand that all of this research has been conducted using pure, refined, synthetic hypericin—not just by grinding up a plant pulled up out of the ground. Research-grade hypericin is the active compound found in the plant, minus the other medicinal compounds found in the herb or the added herbs found in many health food store preparations.

Therefore, the extracts, pills, and potions containing St. John's wort on sale in your local natural foods store may not have the same effect as the research-grade hypericin. It may be less effective—or more effective because of the other active compounds not present in the synthetic research product.

Moreover, research studies tend to use high doses of hypericin, between two and seven times stronger than the doses used to treat depression. This means that it is much more likely to cause side effects.

CONDITIONS HELPED BY ST. JOHN'S WORT

Burns and Wounds

The world's earliest herbalists knew what modern scientists are only just now rediscovering: St. John's wort can speed the healing process, reduce inflammation, and ease pain at the site of injury. Some experts say the plant is especially useful in treating crushed or bruised soft tissue, joints, and nerve endings, helping them heal without infection. It can also take the sting out of minor burns (including sunburn)— which is interesting, given that overdoses of St. John's wort have been linked to phototoxicity. Its success as a popular wound healer may be due in part to its broad action, preventing infection and balancing the immune system as it reduces inflammation and bleeding.

If you use the plant for first-aid purposes, it can be applied directly to the injury as a salve, tincture, or oil infusion, or the tincture can be given orally.

Bacterial Infections

Since ancient times, St. John's wort has been mashed and crumbled and applied on the surface of the skin to prevent infection. Back in the seventeenth century, English herbalist-physician Nicholas Culpeper recommended St. John's wort as a cure for "spitting blood" (tuberculosis). Modern scientists have found that the herb is, in fact, a natural antibiotic that is effective against some of the world's most virulent bacteria. It contains hyperforin and novoimanine, two antibiotic compounds that not only kill bacteria but stimulate the immune system to fight off the infection. An Italian study found that hypericum extract showed a broad antimicrobial activity against both gram-negative and gram-positive bacteria in the test tube.

St. John's wort has been found to be as effective as many of the more traditional drugs, including the sulfonamides (a group of antibiotics commonly prescribed for treatment of bacterial infections). It is also effective against the bacteria that cause strep throat, and can be used to prevent or treat urinary tract infections, ear infections, and colitis as well. Extracts of St. John's wort are known to inhibit the growth of *Mycobacterium tuberculosis,* the most common cause of TB, as well as the bacteria shigella and *Escherichia coli.* St. John's wort also can inhibit the growth of some strains of bacteria that are highly resistant to antibiotics, such as enterococcus, *Pseudomonas aeruginosa,* and *Staphylococcus aureus*, the type of deadly staph infection implicated in modern hospital-related infections. It's effective against bacteria and fungi as well, including the yeast *Candida albicans.*

Viruses

St. John's wort has also shown encouraging promise in treating a wide variety of viruses and retroviruses known as lipid-enveloped viruses— including AIDS, Epstein-Barr virus, influenza, herpes, and viral hepatitis (B and C). Exactly how hypericin fights viruses isn't understood. It may work by inactivating the virus particles, or by hardening the outer surface of the virus so that it can't infect other cells. It may inhibit the reproduction of viruses, especially if administered in the early stages of disease. Indeed, the herb appears to be a "broad spectrum viricidal agent," according to Daniel Meruelo, Ph.D., professor of pathology at NYU.

Researchers from NYU and the Weizmann Institute of Science in Israel reported in the *Journal Proceedings of the National Academy of Sciences* that they discovered two substances in St. John's wort, hypericin and pseudohypericin, that displayed antiviral activity against some retroviruses. Exactly how the antiviral activities occur isn't known, but their chemical structures suggest that they may interact with the viruses' membranes that eventually inactivate the virus.

A European study showed that hypericin has strong antiviral activity in the test tube against herpes simplex virus types I and II (HSV-1 and HSV-2), flu virus, and others. A Japanese study found that a hypericum extract showed antiviral activity against Epstein-Barr virus in the test tube. Other studies suggest that hypericin has an antiviral effect against murine CMV (cytomegalovirus); however, murine CMV is not identical to human CMV, so it isn't known whether hypericin is effective against human CMV.

AIDS and Hepatitis

For more than 10 years, researchers at the New York University Medical Center have been studying hypericin, the most important active compound in St. John's wort. Together with scientists at the Weizmann Institute of Science in Israel, NYU researchers found that hypericin and its cousin pseudohypericin strongly inhibited viruses, including HIV and inactivated HIV in lab tests, preventing infection of new cells. Because this application of hypericin was tried in very preliminary "test-tube" research only, it has not yet been widely tested in humans.

Some of the most exciting work has focused on the role that hypericin might play in the fight against AIDS. So far, early studies have been promising, but experts caution that it is too early to define the depth of the plant's role in treating this dread disease. Researchers are currently investigating hypericin as an adjunct to other AIDS drugs that do suppress HIV production. The research suggests that hypericin appears to be effective in interfering with viruses in four stages of their replication—especially in the first stage, when it renders the virus unable to infect healthy host cells. St. John's wort appears to have the ability to target new viruses as they enter the host and prevent them from infecting host cells. The herb's antiviral properties appear to be more effective in the presence of light. In the test tube, hypericin blocks HIV's ability to form giant cells, which may be one way HIV spreads in the body. Scientists have found that hypericin works in a different way against AIDS than many of the current drugs, including AZT. This could mean that if hypericin works in the body as it does in the test tube, then new combinations of drugs with the plant might attack the virus at two different sites. In fact, one study does show that AZT in combination with hypericin is more effective in curing mice of the friend virus (FV), which is similar to HIV.

New York scientists are also investigating whether hypericin can be used to protect against the spread of virus through blood transfusions. By adding hypericin to a unit of blood, scientists seem to be able to inactivate the virus in that blood.

In the wake of these reports coming from NYU, several American doctors interested in unorthodox AIDS treatments began giving their AIDS patients a standard extract of St. John's wort. In one anecdotal report of just four AIDS patients, two "regained strength" and had an increase in T cell counts (suggesting an improvement in immune function) after taking St. John's wort. However, experts caution that more study is needed before the plant—and the hypericin it contains—can be considered effective against AIDS.

Tests of therapeutic use in animals found that when given right after injection with certain strains of leukemia virus, hypericin completely blocked the disease. Combining hypericin with the AIDS drug AZT appears to result in a virus-fighting drug stronger than either medication alone. The exact antiviral mechanism behind this combination is not known, but scientists do know that the herb works in a different way than AZT.

No human study of antiviral effects of hypericin have been published, and researchers caution AIDS patients not to rush out and purchase St. John's wort as a way to cure the virus. Scientists at NYU have found only minute amounts of hypericin in commercial preparations of St. John's wort. Anyone who does use St. John's wort for HIV should understand that there is no documented research experience with such use in humans, and that serious questions remain about whether commercial preparations of hypericin are effective at all against the virus.

In other research, scientists are currently studying whether St. John's wort may be effective against the hepatitis C virus, a sometimes fatal version of the hepatitis virus that can sometimes lead to cirrhosis and liver cancer. Currently infecting about 150,000 new patients a year, hepatitis C is known as a silent killer because it may cause few symptoms until the disease has destroyed the patient's liver, between 20 and 50 years after initial infection. Researchers at the Bronx VA Hospital and the Mount Sinai Medical Center in New York are treating 24 hepatitis C patients with hypericin.

A San Francisco study inadvertently discovered that St. John's wort appeared to trigger improvements in liver tests of those who had hepatitis. However, liver tests often fluctuate in hepatitis cases, so more study is needed.

Immunity Problems

Herbalists recommend St. John's wort as a powerful boost to the immune system, pointing to its ability to decrease the production of interleukins, a type of messenger that allows immune system cells to communicate with each other. (*Inter* means "between," and *leukin* refers to "white blood cells.") Excessive amounts of interleukins can break down the immune system; as the level of interleukins begins to fall, the body's immune system balances itself. Interestingly, people who are depressed often have very high levels of interleukins; this may be one reason why depressed people have poorly functioning immune systems and, hence, more infections, colds, and other illnesses. Some scientists believe that the experience of depression itself may be related to excessive amounts of interleukins.

Menstrual Problems

St. John's wort is also a popular "women's tonic," capable of easing the pain of both menstrual cramps and premenstrual syndrome

(PMS). An effective painkiller, St. John's wort is said to be an effective treatment for menstrual pain, according to anecdotal reports. Menstrual cramps are caused by high levels of chemicals in the uterus called prostaglandins. Normally, prostaglandins regulate menstrual flow; as a result, high levels of this chemical can cause excessive bleeding, inflammation, or painful uterine contractions—cramps.

Skin Conditions

Because of the plant's ability to respond to light, scientists have been intrigued about whether St. John's wort could treat conditions of the skin. When exposed to light, hypericin becomes highly active and more effective against viruses. This could mean that patients infected with a virus could get a better response from hypericin if they expose themselves to sunlight while taking the herb. Other studies planned to begin in late 1997 will investigate the use of hypericin against warts and other viral skin problems.

At the same time, we know that *too much* St. John's wort can lead to hypersensitivity to the sun (phototoxicity). As a way around this problem, researchers at Iowa State University have isolated the light-giving compound luciferase from fireflies (the light-giving property of the insects) and used it to activate hypericin in the dark. These scientists suggest that patients with viral infections might be able to take a combination of hypericin and luciferase for a stronger antiviral response.

Bedwetting

St. John's wort is indicated in the treatment of children who suffer from bedwetting, according to herbalists. Exactly how this is accomplished is not known.

Cancer

Preliminary studies suggest that St. John's wort may be effective against cancer cells, stopping them from growing when given in low doses, and killing them outright when combined with light therapy in higher doses.

Scientists at the Catholic University in Leuven, Belgium, have found that the herb's hypericin may be helpful in photodynamic therapy, which is used to render tumor tissues more vulnerable to radiation. In the study, scientists injected mice with tumor cells and then divided the animals into two groups. One group got hypericin followed by radiation at the site of tumor injection. The other group received radiation, but no hypericin. As expected, tumors appeared in the control group, but no tumors grew in the mice treated with the hypericin/radiation combo. Moreover, the radiation had no toxic effect on the rat's normal skin next to the tumor.

It's also possible that the herb may be a safe, effective alternative in the treatment of melanoma (a particularly deadly form of skin cancer) and glioma (a type of brain tumor), according to studies at several U.S. universities. A hypericum oil extract inhibited growth of tumors and increased body weight in rats.

St. John's wort is being used to treat six severely ill glioma patients who have not responded to any other medicine at Trinity Medical Center in North Dakota. Some researchers noted that the action of the herb appeared to be very similar to the cancer drug tamoxifen, one of the most widely used breast cancer drugs. The hypericin in the study is purified, synthetic hypericin. While it's too soon to tell results, the patients have tolerated the dosage (in escalating doses) well.

Other studies at UCLA are looking at how well hypericum can attack other kinds of cancers, including breast cancer and melanoma.

In addition to treating cancer, St. John's wort may work to prevent malignancy as well, according to one study published in a 1993 issue of *Basic Life Sciences*. In that report, hypericum extract prevented cellular DNA from mutating after radiation damage—the preliminary stage of cancer. In other studies, the herb shows some protective ability against radiation damage to intestinal linings and bone marrow.

Stomach Irritations

Folk healers have used the blossoms of St. John's wort to ease ulcers, gastritis, diarrhea, and nausea. It has a favorable action on the secretion of bile, soothing the digestive system.

Other Conditions

Herbalists also give out St. John's wort to treat insomnia, jaundice, headache, anemia, pulmonary complaints, bladder troubles, dysentery, worms, and inflammations of the nose and throat.

CHAPTER 9

Finding an Alternative Health Care Provider

Nearly 80 percent of the world's population uses herbal medicine—but the United States is not one of those places that has yet fully embraced the practice. And yet many of our medicines were derived from plant sources—with many more possibilities out there, if we only took the time to look. Botanists believe there may be as many as 500,000 plants on earth today, but only about 5,000 of them have been extensively studied for their medicinal properties. More than 121 of our best prescription drugs come from only 90 species of plants—and 74 percent of these plant-based drugs were discovered by investigating the ancient claims of well-trained herbalists. It's logical to suspect that the plant world may well harbor many more medicinal treasures yet to be unearthed.

Although herbal medicine makes up a large part of what is practiced as "traditional" medicine elsewhere in the world, since the 1930s the practice of medicine in the United States has focused almost completely on a strict science-based system, excluding any alternative type of treatment.

Yet today, of the 119 plant-derived pharmaceutical medicines, about 75 percent are still used in ways similar to those traditionally practiced by native peoples, according to the World Health Organization. About 25 percent of all our prescription drugs are still derived directly from trees, shrubs, or herbs.

Inexplicably, modern U.S. medicine has generally turned its back on using pure herbs in treating disease. One of the reasons has been financial, since herbs cannot be patented, and drug companies can't hold the exclusive right to sell a plant—therefore, companies have not been motivated to invest money in herbal testing or promotion. Moreover, collecting and preparing herbs for medicine isn't as easily controlled as is the manufacturing process for producing synthetic drugs. Furthermore, many of these plants grow in places both distant and unstable, making it difficult to obtain a ready supply. And as Americans have come to rely on commercial drugs to provide quick relief despite the severe side effects, they have come to view herbs—with few side effects—as weak and ineffective.

Slowly, the viewpoint appears to be changing. In the wake of a review of European studies pointing to the efficacy of St. John's wort and depression, more and more physicians are incorporating alternative types of treatment in their practices—or at least not disapproving when their patients come to them for approval of an unorthodox treatment.

HOW HERBS WORK

There are a large number of active compounds in plants that have biological activity. Chemists have been trying to isolate and purify them for the past 150 years. Herbs that have already yielded valuable compounds for synthetic drugs include reserpine from *Rauwolfia serpentina* (Indian snakeroot), digoxin from *Digitalis purpurea* (foxglove), morphine from *Papaver somniafera* (opium poppy), colchicine from *Colchicum autumnale* (autumn crocus), and so on.

Unlike their synthetic cousins, herbs have an effect on the human body that is generally slower and gentler, because they must use an indirect way of getting to the bloodstream and certain organs. (Of course, this isn't always true, and the wrong herb can cause toxic effects if used incorrectly or in the wrong amount.)

HERBAL MEDICINE

The practice of herbal medicine is not regulated or licensed in the United States. As a result, herbalists practice outside the boundaries of the traditional health care system. Experts in the science of herbs may use approaches based on an Asian approach (such as Chinese medicine or the Indian system of Ayurveda), or they may be naturopathic physicians.

Traditional Chinese medicine emphasizes the restoration of harmony, as expressed in the five elements (fire, earth, metal, water, and wool) and two complementary forces—yin and yang. Herbs are an important part of this balance. Ayurvedic medicine is rooted in the ancient Indian culture, and also recognizes five elements—ether, fire, water, air, and earth. Ayurvedic physicians try to balance the elements of air or wind, fire or bile, and water or phlegm, and employ herbs in this effort. Even in Western medicine, most drug groups were developed from the plant kingdom, although they may be produced synthetically now.

In order to help you find qualified help in herbal medicine, there are a wide variety of organizations (see Appendices D and K) from which to choose.

NATUROPATHY

Naturopathic medicine treats health conditions by using the body's inborn ability to heal itself, using a variety of alternative methods based on the patient's needs. Naturopathic doctors stress the importance of healing the person, not the disease. Methods may include nutrition counseling, herbal medicine, homeopathy, acupuncture, hydrotherapy, physical medicine, counseling, lifestyle moderation, and minor surgery.

Naturopathy is especially good at treating chronic illness, where traditional medicine has not succeeded. Many experts recommend consulting a traditional physician for a diagnosis, and then going to see a naturopathic physician for treatment.

Seven states license naturopathic physicians in the United States: Alaska, Arizona, Connecticut, Hawaii, Montana, Oregon, and Washington, and in five Canadian provinces: Alberta, British Columbia, Manitoba, Ontario, and Saskatchewan. At present, several other states are considering their own licensing provisions. Accredited colleges of naturopathic medicine include the Bastyr University in Seattle, the National College of Naturopathic Medicine in Portland, the Southwest College in Scottsdale, AZ, and the Canadian College of Naturopathic Medicine in Etobicoke, Ontario.

Unfortunately, only a few insurance companies will reimburse you for the services of a naturopathic physician.

Where to Buy Hypericum Extract

While St. John's wort is sold in a variety of forms, most herbalists believe that you'll get the best results by using the same type of hypericum that is used in scientific studies. Usually referred to as LI 160 in research articles (German brand name Jarsin or Jarsin 300), this formulation is available by mail and retail in the United States and Canada. The most effective formulation is 300 mg of *Hypericum perforatum*, standardized at 0.3 percent hypericin.

Canada

Canadians can buy St. John's wort from U.S. suppliers. However, here is a source for those who want to buy from a Canadian supplier:
Health Service Center
971 Bloor Street West
Toronto, Ontario 46H 1L7
(416) 535-9562

United Kingdom

Baldwin's
173 Walworth Road
London SE 17 1RW
44-0171-703-5550

United States

Eclectic Institute
Sandy, OR 97055
(800) 332-4372
Organic, hypoallergenic, and made without corn or grain alcohol. Best choice for those allergic to corn or grains. Available in black cherry or plain, with vitamin C.

Elixir Tonics & Teas
8612 Melrose Avenue
West Hollywood, CA 90069
(888) 486-6427
Vegi-cap capsules (made with no animal products), called "St. John's wort whole extract."

Gaia Herbs
Harvard, MA 01451
(800) 831-7780
St. John's wort extracted from
flowers and buds only.

Herb Pharm
Williams, OR 97544
(800) 348-4372
St. John's wort extracted from
flowers and buds only.

Hypericum Buyers Club
8205 Santa Monica Boulevard
Suite 472
Los Angeles, CA 90046
(888) 497-3742 (toll-free 24 hours)
Standardized capsules (Hypericum
Verbatim) of the same type used
in depression studies.

McZand Herbal
P.O. Box 5312
Santa Monica, CA 90409
(800) 800-0405
More concentrated (and more ex-
pensive) than most.

Nature's Answer
Hauppage, NY 11788
Not sold directly to the public; can
be ordered through natural food
stores. Kosher and alcohol-free extract. Strict vegetarians may want
to choose this product, since it is
made with vegetable glycerin (not
animal glycerin).

Nature's Plus
548 Broadhollow Road
Melville, NY 11747
(800) 645-9500
Standardized extract made with
vegetable glycerin.

Planetary Formulations
P.O. Box 533
Soquel, CA 95073
(800) 776-7701
Very concentrated extract (more so
than most).

Standardized Brands Available at Stores

"Kira"
Lichtwer Pharma US, Inc.
Sugar-coated tablets available at
drugstores and department stores.

"St. John's wort"
Enzymatic Therapy
Gelatin capsules available at
health food stores.

"St. John's wort"
Nature's Resources
Gelatin capsules available at
drugstores and mass markets.

"St. John's wort"
Solaray
"Guaranteed potency" gelatin
capsule (300 mg) available at
health food stores.

Seed Suppliers

You can buy seeds to grow your own St. John's wort. The following companies are among those that offer seeds:

Seeds of Change
P.O. Box 15700
Santa Fe, NM 87506
(888) 762-7333
Offers organic St. John's wort seeds (heirloom variety); 100 seeds for $2.29 plus postage.

Seed Savers Exchange
3076 North Winn Road
Decorah, IA 52101
(319) 382-5872
Membership of $7 a year allows you to buy heirloom St. John's wort seeds from other members.

Herbal Associations

Canada

Canadian Association of Ayurvedic
Medicine
P.O. Box 749 Station B
Ottawa, Ontario K1P 5P8
(613) 837-5737
Maintains a list of Canadian
Ayurvedic doctors and supports
research.

Ontario Herbalists' Association
7 Alpine Avenue
Toronto, Ontario M6P 3R6
(416) 536-1509

United States

Alternative Medical Association
7909 Southeast State Street
Portland, OR 97215
(503) 254-7555

American Association of Acupuncture and Oriental Medicine
4101 Lake Boone Trail, Suite 201
Raleigh, NC 27607
(919) 787-5181

This national professional trade
organization of acupuncturists who
meet acceptable standards can provide you with names of local
members.

American Association of Naturopathic Physicians
2366 Eastlake Avenue East,
Suite 322
Seattle, WA 98102
(206) 827-6035
For $5 you can get brochures on
naturopathic medicine and a list
of licensed naturopaths in the
United States. Publishes a quarterly newsletter for professionals
and lay readers.

American Botanical Council
P.O. Box 201660
Austin, TX 78720
(512) 331-8868
Nonprofit research and education
organization. Publishes *Herbal-
Gram* magazine, herb booklets,
and reprints of scientific articles.

American Herb Association
P.O. Box 353
Rescue, CA 96672
Publishes a newsletter covering a wide range of herbal topics.

The American Herbalists Guild
P.O. Box 1683
Sequel, CA 95073
Offers a directory of schools and teachers.

American Herbal Products
Association
P.O. Box 2410
Austin, TX 78768

American Holistic Medical
Association
4101 Lake Boone Trail, Suite 201
Raleigh, NC 27607
(919) 787-5146
Provides a list of holistic physicians in the United States for $5.

Herb Research Foundation
1007 Pearl Street, Suite 200
Boulder, CO 80302
(303) 449-2265

International Herb Growers and
Marketers Association
1202 Allanson Road
Mundeleiin, IL 60060

Helpful Publications

*American Herb Association
Newsletter*
P.O. Box 353
Rescue, CA 96672
One of the oldest herb newsletters.

Botanical and Herb Reviews
B&H Reviews
P.O. Box 106
Eureka Springs, AK 72632
Quarterly publication.

Canadian Journal of Herbalism
11 Winthrop Place
Stoney Creek, Ontario L8G 3M3

The Herb Companion
201 East Fourth Street
Loveland, CO 80537

HerbalGram
American Botanical Council
P.O. Box 201660
Austin, TX 78720
(800) 373-7105
Quarterly magazine of the
Botanical Council and the Herb
Research Foundation.

*Journal of Herbs, Spices and
Medicinal Plants*
Haworth Press
10 Alice Street
Binghamton, NY 13904

Medical Herbalism
Bergner Communications
P.O. Box 33080
Portland, OR 97233
(503) 242-9815
Published six times a year.

Web Sites for St. John's Wort and Depression

Dr. Weil Web site
http://cgi.pathfinder.com/drweil
Search the archives for
information on St. John's wort.

Herb Central "Herb of the Month"
http://www.the.net/rtanner/herb-oct.htm
This commercial site still offers a
good discussion of St. John's wort,
in addition to products and handy
links to other sites.

Herb Forum Room
http://www.mothernature.com/
wwwboard/herbs/index.htm

Herbal Information Center
http://gic.simplenet.com/dr/herb/
stjohn.htm
Links to books, transcript of *20/20*
show on St. John's wort, and
more.

Herbal remedies
http://www.all-natural.com/
hyp-1.html
Herbal remedies for depression.

*Hypericin-St. John's Wort
Information Sheet*
http://www.thebody.com/.../pwa/
hyper.html
Information on St. John's wort as
a potential treatment for AIDS.

The Hypericum Home Page
http://www.hypericum.com
A site dedicated to information
about St. John's wort and offering
a consortium of vendors.

Medicinal herb FAQ
http://sunsite.unc.edu/herbmed/
mediher1.html#c2-1-4

Medicine net
http://www.medicinenet.com/
mainmenu/news/depress.htm
Information and links about
depression.

Mental health net
http://www.cmhc.com/articles/
depress.1.htm
Information about depression and
treatments.

Natural living
http://www.healthyideas.com/
healing/herb/stjohn.html
Herbal remedies and information
on natural living.

*Natural Prozac Program: How to
Use St. John's Wort*
http://www.all-natural.com/
natproz3.htm
Information on St. John's wort.

St. John's wort
http://www.botanical.com/
botanical/mgmh/s/sajohn06.html
Links to detailed information
about hypericum.

St. John's wort
http://www.kcweb.com/herb/
stjohn.htm
This handy informational site is a
commercial Web site but offers
straightforward details.

*St. John's wort: herbal relief for
depression*
http://www.all-natural.com/
hyp25.htm

*St. John's Wort: Why All the
Attention?*
http://www.health-pages.com/sj/
sj.html
Information about what conditions
it treats, links to other sites, and a
bibliography.

St. John's wort personal experience
http://www.canuck.com/kelm/
stjohns.html

Quiz: Are You Depressed?

- Do you feel very sad or cry a great deal?

- Have you gained or lost weight? Do you binge or overeat?

- Do you have chronic insomnia or excessive sleepiness? Are you tired all the time, no matter how much sleep you get?

- Do you have outbursts of complaints or shouting? Do you feel resentful and angry?

- Have you lost interest in hobbies or activities that you used to enjoy?

- Have you lost interest in sex?

- Do you feel worthless, unattractive, or inappropriately guilty?

- Do you have a hard time concentrating? Are your thoughts muddy or foggy?

- Do you brood? Do you have phobias, delusions, or fears?

- Do you have trouble sitting still?

- Do you have slowed body movements and speech?

- Have you thought you'd be better off dead?

If you answered "yes" to three or more of these symptoms, you may want to consult a mental health expert.

Warning Signs of Impending Suicide

Someone thinking about suicide may exhibit one or more of the following signs. Anyone showing suicidal signs should be encouraged to seek professional help as soon as possible. Take all threats seriously—it is not true that someone who threatens suicide will not follow through.

- *Withdrawal.* Someone contemplating suicide may feel an overwhelming urge to be alone, an unwillingness to communicate, or a desire to withdraw into a shell. Trouble with grades or job performance can signal such a retreat.

- *Life crisis.* Death, divorce, job loss, or accident can trigger suicide in a deeply depressed person.

- *Behavior change.* Changes in appearance, energy, or attitude can be an outward sign of suicidal thoughts.

- *Aggression.* A suicidal person may have a sudden interest in dangerous pursuits, sports, or unsafe sexual practices.

- *Mood change.* Sudden calm after severe depression may indicate a person has chosen suicide as a solution to problems.

- *Gift giving.* A suicidal person may suddenly bequeath treasured possessions.

Your Chances of Inheriting Depression

While anyone can become depressed, it is possible to inherit the vulnerability toward developing a serious depression.

- *Relatives.* If a close relative is depressed, you are 15 percent more likely to also inherit major depression.

- *Twins.* If your identical twin is depressed, you're 67 percent more likely to be depressed yourself.

- *Substance abuse.* If your depressed relatives abuse alcohol or drugs as a symptom of their depression, you're 8 to 10 times more likely to do the same.

- *Suicide.* If a close relative has committed suicide, you are likely to commit suicide yourself if you become depressed.

- *Women.* Close female relatives of depressed women have a 1 in 4 chance of inheriting major depression, and a 9 in 10 chance of having mild depression.

Drugs That Can Cause Depression

The following drugs are known to cause depression in some people:

benzodiazepines

bromocriptine

clonidine

cortisone-like steroids

digitalis

Halcion

hormones (estrogen, progesterone, cortisol, prednisone)

indomethacin

levodopa

methyldopa

oral contraceptives

phenothiazines (some)

reserpine

Valium

How to Find an Alternative Health Care Provider

If you want to find a health care provider who can guide you in the use of St. John's wort, your best bet may be to contact one of the organizations listed below for a list of local holistic health care providers in your area.

Canada

Canadian Association of Ayurvedic
Medicine
P.O. Box 749 Station B
Ottawa, Ontario K1P 5P8
(613) 837-5737
Maintains a list of Canadian
Ayurvedic doctors and supports
research.

International College of
Traditional Chinese Medicine
3011847 West Broadway
Vancouver, BC V6M 461
(604) 731-2926

United States

Alternative Medical Association
7909 Southeast State Street
Portland, OR 97215
(503) 254-7555

American Association of
Acupuncture and Oriental
Medicine
4101 Lake Boone Trail, Suite 201
Raleigh, NC 27607
(919) 787-5181
This national professional trade
organization of acupuncturists who
meet acceptable standards can
provide you with names of local
members.

American Association of
Naturopathic Physicians
2366 Eastlake Avenue East,
Suite 322
Seattle, WA 98102
(206) 827-6035
For $5 you can get a list of
licensed naturopaths in the United
States.

The American Herbalists Guild
P.O. Box 1683
Sequel, CA 95073
Offers a directory of teachers.

American Holistic Medical
Association
4101 Lake Boone Trail, Suite 201
Raleigh, NC 27607
(919) 787-5146
Provides a list of holistic
physicians in the United States
for $5.

College of Maharishi
Ayur-Veda Health Center
P.O. Box 282
Fairfield, IA 52556
(515) 472-5866
Provides referrals to health centers
which offer methods for
prevention and treatment of a
broad range of illnesses.

Foundation for the Advancement
of Innovative Medicine
P.O. Box 338
Kinderhook, NY 12106
Organizations of professionals and
lay people that advocates for
holistic and alternative practices,
they are a good source of referrals
in the New York City area.

International Academy of
Nutrition and Preventive Medicine
P.O. Box 18433
Asheville, NC 28814
(704) 258-3243
Serves as a clearinghouse of
information and a referral service
for physicians practicing
orthomolecular medicine

National College of Naturopathic
Medicine
11231 SE Market St.
Portland, OR 97216
(503) 255-4860
Provides a list of naturopathic
doctors in the U.S. and offers a
degree program in naturopathic
medicine.

Recipes for St. John's Wort Oil, Tea, and Tincture

St. John's Wort Oil

1. Grind 1 cup fresh flowers (the fresher the better) to a pulp, or grind dried flowers to a powder.
2. Place in 1-quart canning jar.
3. Pour in extra-virgin olive oil to cover. Let stand in a warm place.
4. Keep jar out of sunlight, and shake every day.
5. After at least 2 weeks, strain through a linen cloth or several layers of cheesecloth, and bottle for use. (The oil should be a deep dark red. If the color is pink, use fresher flowers.)

St. John's Wort Tea

1. Steep 1 teaspoon dried flowers in 1 cup boiling water for 15 minutes.
2. Strain. Drink 1 cup three times a day.

St. John's Wort Tincture

1. Grind 1 cup fresh flowers (the fresher the better) to a pulp, or grind dried flowers to a powder.
2. Place in 1-quart canning jar.
3. Pour in 100-proof vodka to cover. Let stand in a warm place.
4. Keep jar out of sunlight, and shake every day.
5. After at least 2 weeks, strain through a linen cloth or several layers of cheesecloth, and bottle for use. (The oil should be a deep dark red. If the color is pink, use fresher flowers.)

Glossary

amino acids Any organic acid containing one or more amino groups; a basic part of proteins and basic building blocks of neurotransmitters.

Anafranil The brand name for clomipramine, a tricyclic antidepressant that is also prescribed for obsessive-compulsive disorder.

anhedonia The inability to experience pleasure from activities that once brought joy.

antagonist A drug that reduces or blocks the action of another drug.

anticholinergic effects The interference with the action of acetylcholine in the brain and peripheral nervous system by any drug. This term is often used to refer to the side effects of tricyclic antidepressants, such as dry mouth, blurry vision, and constipation.

antidepressant A medication used to treat depression.

anti-inflammatory A substance that soothes inflammation or reduces the inflammatory response of the tissue.

Asendin The brand name for amoxapine, a tricyclic antidepressant.

Ativan The brand name for lorazepam, an antianxiety medication also prescribed for anxiety with depression.

atypical bipolar II depression A clinical condition in which periods of major depression alternate with periods of mild elation.

atypical depression A type of depression in which the person reacts to the environment, is sensitive to rejection, and may gain weight and sleep more than usual. This condition is the opposite of typical depression, characterized by weight loss and insomnia.

Aventyl A brand name for nortriptyline, a tricyclic antidepressant.

barbiturate A habit-forming drug used to induce sleep or treat anxiety.

behavior therapy A form of psychotherapy that seeks to modify behavior by manipulating the environment and behavior.

benzodiazepines A class of drugs that have a hypnotic and sedative action, used mainly as tranquilizers to control symptoms due to anxiety or stress, and as a sleeping aid.

biogenic amine hypothesis The idea that abnormalities in the biogenic amines (especially the neurotransmitters norepinephrine, dopamine, and serotonin) are involved in depression.

biogenic amines Organic substances subdivided into catecholamines (epinephrine, dopamine, and norepinephrine) and indoles (tryptophan and serotonin), all of which appear to play a role in the development of depression.

bipolar disorder A major affective disorder characterized by both depression and mania. A mild form of this disorder is sometimes called cyclothymia. Bipolar disorders may be divided into manic, depressed, or mixed types, on the basis of the patient's symptoms. In manic type, symptoms include excitement, euphoria, expansive or irritable mood, hyperactivity, pressured speech, flight of ideas, limited sleep needs, distractibility, and impaired judgment. There may be grandiose or elated delusions. In depressed type, symptoms include slow thinking, lowered mood, decreased movement or agitation, loss of interest, guilt, negative self-esteem, sleep problems, and appetite loss.

bipolar I disorder Also known as manic-depression, a clinical condition characterized by alternating episodes of major depression and mania or elation, often severe enough to require hospitalization.

bipolar II disorder A clinical condition characterized by alternating periods of major depression and mild mania. A patient may need to be hospitalized during depressed periods, but usually not during the manic phase.

bipolar III disorder A term used to describe a depressed person who develops mild or severe mania only after taking certain drugs (such as antidepressants).

bupropion The generic name for Wellbutrin, an antidepressant drug.

BuSpar The brand name for buspirone, a non-habit-forming antianxiety medication.

buspirone The generic name for BuSpar, a non-habit-forming antianxiety medication.

Candida albicans A small fungus or yeast that is the primary disease-causing organism of the infection moniliasis candidiasis (candida).

carbamazepine The generic name for Tegretol.

clinical depression A medical term often used for major depression.

clomipramine The generic name for Anafranil, a tricyclic antidepressant.

cognitive therapy A structured form of short-term psychotherapy in which the goal is to change the negative, inaccurate ways of thinking.

cortisol A stress hormone, usually referred to as hydrocortisone. Closely related to cortisone in physiological effects.

cyclothymia A form of manic-depression characterized by relatively mild highs and lows.

cytomegalovirus (CMV) A virus related to the herpes virus that inhabits the salivary glands.

Cytomel A thyroid hormone sometimes used to boost the effectiveness of an antidepressant.

decoction The process of boiling hard and woody herbs in water to ensure that their soluble content reaches the water. Herb and water are mixed together, brought to a boil, and allowed to simmer for 10 to 15 minutes.

Depakote The brand name for valproic acid, an anticonvulsant drug and an alternative to lithium for the treatment of manic-depression.

Deprenyl A European monoamine oxidase inhibitor that lacks the "cheese effect" (a harmful interaction with cheese and other tyramine-containing foods); used to treat Parkinson's disease.

depressive illness Endogenous depression characterized by depressed mood, reduced energy level, and poor self-image.

depressive personality disorder A type of depressive disorder in which the essential feature is a pattern of depressive thoughts and behaviors that begins by early adulthood, including dejection, gloominess, cheerlessness, joylessness, and unhappiness. It remains controversial whether the distinction between depressive personality disorder and dysthymic disorder is useful.

depressive reaction A reactive depression that represents an understandable response to a significant loss or stressful life situation, involving despondency and distress. It is usually comparatively mild to moderate, and usually passes within 2 weeks to 6 months.

desipramine The generic name for Norpramin, a tricyclic antidepressant.

Desyrel The brand name for trazodone, an antidepressant structurally unlike the tricyclics, MAOIs, and SSRIs.

diazepam The generic name for Valium.

dopamine One of the major neurotransmitters found in the synapses of the brain. Low levels of dopamine are associated with depression.

dysphoria An unpleasant mood associated with a shifting set of symptoms, including sadness, anxiety, and irritability.

dysthymia A mild but persistent form of depression. Dysthymic disorder (also called "depressive neurosis") is a mild, chronic disturbance of mood involving depression that lasts for at least two years. Other symptoms include poor appetite or overeating, insomnia or excessive fatigue, low energy, poor self-esteem, poor concentration, or hopelessness. The mild depression does not last long enough, or is not severe enough, to meet the criteria for a diagnosis of major depression.

Effexor The brand name for venlafaxine, an antidepressant.

Elavil The brand name for amitriptyline, a tricyclic antidepressant.

endocrine gland A gland that secretes directly into the bloodstream.

endogenous depression A spontaneous, unexplained, and seemingly unprovoked depression of moderate to severe degree.

endorphins Natural opiates produced in the brain which function as the body's own natural painkillers.

enzyme Any one of the numerous complex proteins that are produced by living cells and catalyze specific biochemical reactions.

epinephrine Also known as adrenaline, one of the catecholamines secreted by the adrenal gland and the sympathetic nervous system responsible for physical symptoms of fear and anxiety.

fluoxetine The generic name for Prozac, an SSRI antidepressant.

fluvoxamine The generic name for Luvox, an SSRI antidepressant.

GABA The common abbreviation for the term gamma-aminobutyric acid, a neurotransmitter that controls the flow of nerve impulses by blocking the release of other neurotransmitters.

generic drugs A drug not controlled by a manufacturer's trademark, and usually sold more cheaply than a brand name.

Halcion The brand name for triazolam, a short-acting benzodiazepine hypnotic or sleeping pill.

hypericin The primary active compound in the plant hypericum (St. John's wort) thought to be related to the plant's antidepressant action.

hypericum The formal name for the plant commonly known as St. John's wort, of the genus *Hypericum.*

hyperthymia A mood characterized by high energy, confidence, and activity, more energetic than a normal mood but less so than in mild forms of mania.

hypomania A mildly elevated mood lasting a few days, less intense than mania but more intense than hyperthymia.

hypothalamus A part of the brain responsible for regulating automatic activities of the body, including hunger, thirst, sleep, body temperature, and sexual activity.

imipramine The generic name for Tofranil, a tricyclic antidepressant.

infusion The simplest method of preparing an herb tea, using either fresh or dried herbs. Herbs are mixed with boiling water, covered, and steeped for 5 to 10 minutes. Infusions may be taken hot, cold, or iced.

interleukin A compound produced by the body in response to infection, inflammation, or other challenges.

isocarboxazid The generic name for Marplan, an antidepressant MAO inhibitor.

leukocytes White blood cells.

levodopa The precursor of dopamine.

lithium An element that, when used as a medication, can stabilize fluctuating ups and downs of mood disorders by shifting the levels of water and electrolytes.

L-tryptophan An amino acid used to make serotonin.

Ludiomil The brand name for maprotiline, a tetracyclic antidepressant.

Luvox The brand name for fluvoxamine, an SSRI antidepressant.

major affective disorder A group of disorders with a persistent, prominent disturbance of mood (depression or mania) and a full syndrome of symptoms. Major depression and bipolar disorder are both examples of major affective disorder.

major depressive episode Also known as clinical or unipolar depression, or major depressive disorder, an episode lasting at least 2 weeks, characterized by at least four of the following symptoms: loss of ability to experience pleasure and interest, fatigue, feelings of worthlessness or guilt, concen-

tration problems, appetite and sleep disturbances, and frequent thoughts of suicide and death.

mania A period of persistent elation characterized by hyperactivity, agitation, rapid talking, excitement, or flight of ideas.

manic-depressive illness A disorder characterized by alternating episodes of moderate to severe depression and unstable periods of elation. It is also known as bipolar I disorder. The periods of mania are distinct, with a predominant mood that is expansive or irritable. Other symptoms include hyperactivity, flight of ideas, inflated self-esteem, little need for sleep, distractibility, and excessive involvement in activities that may be flamboyant, bizarre, or disorganized.

MAOI The abbreviation for monoamine oxidase inhibitor, a type of antidepressant.

maprotiline The generic name for Ludiomil, a tetracyclic antidepressant.

Marplan The brand name for isocarboxazid, an MAOI.

MHPG A major metabolite of norepinephrine excreted in urine. Low levels occur in depression, while high levels are found in bipolar patients during manic phases. Research suggests that MHPG levels may be used to classify depression types and to predict responses to tricyclic antidepressants.

monoamine oxidase (MAO) An enzyme that breaks down neurotransmitters. Inhibiting this enzyme by certain antidepressant drugs (MAO inhibitors) may ease a patient's depression.

monoamine oxidase inhibitors (MAOIs) A class of antidepressants that keeps the enzyme monoamine oxidase from breaking down neurotransmitters, resulting in higher levels of norepinephrine and serotonin at the nerve synapses.

mood (affective) disorders A group of clinical conditions characterized by feelings of lack of control over mood or emotions, primarily depression and mania. Mood disorders can affect basic functions, such as cognitive ability, sleep patterns, appetite, and sexuality, and can interfere with personal and professional life.

Nardil The brand name for phenelzine, an MAOI.

nefazadone The generic name for the antidepressant Serzone.

neurotransmitter A chemical in the nervous system (such as serotonin or dopamine) that carries messages across the gaps between neurons. Dysfunction of this neurotransmitter system has been linked to depression.

norepinephrine Also called noradrenaline, one of the three major neurotransmitters found in the brain and implicated in the development of depression. High levels of norepinephrine have been linked to manic states; low levels, to depression.

norfluoxetine A metabolite of Prozac.

Norpramin The brand name for desipramine, a tricyclic antidepressant.

nortriptyline The generic name for the tricyclic antidepressants Pamelor and Aventyl.

obsessive compulsive disorder A clinical condition characterized by distressing repetition of thoughts that are intense, frightening, absurd or unusual, together with ritualized actions that are usually bizarre and irrational.

orthostatic hypotension A precipitous fall in blood pressure upon sitting or standing up, causing dizziness or fainting. This is a common side effect in some antidepressants.

Pamelor The brand name for nortriptyline, a tricyclic antidepressant.

Parnate The brand name for tranylcypromine, an MAOI antidepressant.

paroxetine The generic name for Paxil, an SSRI antidepressant.

Paxil The brand name for paroxetine, an SSRI antidepressant.

phototoxic Refers to injury by ultraviolet radiation or light.

placebo Substances having no pharmacological effect; a "dummy" pill.

protriptyline The generic name for Vivactil, a tricyclic antidepressant.

Prozac The brand name for fluoxetine, an SSRI antidepressant.

psychotropic drugs Medications that affect mood or mental activity.

seasonal affective disorder (SAD) A mood disorder characterized by mental depression related to a certain season of the year (usually winter), including day-

time drowsiness, fatigue, and diminished concentration. It is four times more common in women.

selective serotonin reuptake inhibitors (SSRIs) A class of antidepressants that work by blocking the reabsorption of serotonin in the brain, raising the levels of serotonin. SSRIs include Prozac, Zoloft, and Paxil.

serotonin One of the three major types of neurotransmitters found in the synapses of the brain linked to the development of depression.

sertraline The generic name for Zoloft, an SSRI antidepressant.

Serzone The brand name for nefazadone, a serotonin-related antidepressant similar to an SSRI.

SSRI Selective serotonin reuptake inhibitor.

subclinical depression A form of depression not severe enough to meet the diagnostic criteria for major depression or dysthymia.

Surmontil The brand name for trimipramine, a tricyclic antidepressant.

synapse The gap between two nerve cells at which the transmission of nerve impulses occur.

Tegretol The brand name for carbamazepine, an anticonvulsant drug used as an alternative to lithium for the treatment of manic-depression.

tetracyclic A class of antidepressants named for their four-ring chemical structure. Ludiomil is an example of a tetracyclic.

Tofranil The brand name for imipramine, the first tricyclic antidepressant.

tranylcypromine The generic name for Parnate, an MAOI antidepressant.

trazodone The generic name for Desyrel, an antidepressant.

tricyclic antidepressants (TCAs) A class of antidepressants named for their three-ring chemical structure. TCAs increase the level of norepinephrine and serotonin in the synapses of the brain.

unipolar disorder Recurrent major depression.

valproic acid The generic name for Depakote, an anticonvulsive medicine to treat manic-depression.

venlafaxine The generic name for Effexor, an SSRI.

Vivactil The brand name for protriptyline, a tricyclic antidepressant.

Wellbutrin The brand name for bupropion, an antidepressant with a structure unlike SSRIs, MAOIs, or tricyclics.

Zoloft The brand name for sertraline, an SSRI antidepressant.

References

Akerele, O., "WHO guidelines for the assessment of herbal medicines," *Fitoterapia* 62 (1992) 99–110; summarized in *HerbalGram* 28 (1993) 13–20.

AIDS Weekly Plus staff, "Herbal medicine: Pharmaceutical versions developed," *AIDS Weekly Plus* (Feb. 24, 1997) 11–12.

Barbagallo, C., and Chisare, G., "Antimicrobial activity of three hypericum species," *Fitoterapia* 58/3 (1987) 175–177.

Barnard, D. L., et al., "Evaluation of the antiviral activity of anthraquinones, anthrones, and anthraquinone derivatives against human cytomegalovirus," *Antiviral Research* 17/1 (1992) 63–77.

Bender, K. J., "St. John's wort evaluated as herbal antidepressant," *Mental Health Source* (online http://www.mhsource.com) (Oct. 1996).

Bergmann, R., Nubner, J., and Deming, J., "Behandlung leichter bis mittelschwerer Depressionen," *Therapiewoch Neurologie/Psychiatrie* 7/23 (1993) 5–40.

Bisset, N. G. (ed.), *Herbal Drugs and Phytopharmaceuticals* (Stuttgart: Medpharm Scientific, 1994).

Bladt, S., and Wagner, H., "Inhibition of MAO by fractions of and constituents of hypericum extract," *Geriatric Psychiatry and Neurology* 7 suppl. 1 (1994) S57–59.

Bombardelli, E., and Morazzoni, P., "*Hypericum perforatum*," *Fitoterapia* 62/1 (1995) 43–68.

Burton Goldberg group, *Alternative Medicine: The Definitive Guide* (Fife, WA: Future Medicine, 1995).

Castleman, M., *The Healing Herbs* (Emmaus, PA: Rodale Press, 1991).

Cott, J., "Natural product formulations available in Europe for psychotropic indications," *Psychopharmacology Bulletin* 31 (1995) 745–751.

De Smet, P. A., "Should herbal medicine-like products be licensed as medicines?" *British Medical Journal* 310 (1995) 1023–1027.

————, "St. John's wort as an antidepressant" (editorial), *British Medical Journal* 313 (1996) 241–247.

Ditzler, K., Gessner, B., Schatton, W., and Willems, A. S., "Clinical trial on Neuropas versus placebo in patients with mild to moderate depressive symptoms: A placebo controlled, randomized double blind study," *Complementary Therapies in Medicine* 2 (1994) 5–13.

Ernst, E., "St. John's wort, an antidepressant—a systematic, criteria-based review," *Phytomedicine* 2/1 (1995) 67–71.

Foster, S., "Fighting depression the herbal way," *Herbs for Health* (Nov./Dec. 1996) 51–53.

Hahn, G., "*Hypericum perforatum*—a medicinal herb used in antiquity and still of interest today," *Journal of Naturopathic Medicine* 3/1 (1992) 94–96.

Halama, P., "Wirksamkeit des Johanniskraut extraktes LI 160 bei depressiver Versrimmung," *Nervenheilkunde* 10 (1991) 250–253.

Hansgen, K., and Vesper, J., "Antidepressive Wirksamkeit eines hochdosierten Hypericum-extraktes," *Munch Med Wschr* 138 (1996) 35–43.

Hansgen, K., Vesper, J., and Ploch, M., "Multicenter double blind study examining the antidepressant effectiveness of the hypericum extract LI 160," *Journal of Geriatric Psychiatry and Neurology* 7 suppl. 1 (1994) S15–18.

Harrer, G., Hubner, W., and Podzuweit, H., "Effectiveness and tolerance of the hypericum extract LI 160 compared to maprotiline: A multicenter double blind study," *Journal of Geriatric Psychiatry and Neurology* 7 suppl. 1 (1994) S24–28.

Harrer, G., Schmidt, U., and Khun, U., "Alternative Depressions behandlung mit einum Hypericum-Extract," *Therapieworch Neurologie/Psychuatrie* 5 (1991) 710–716.

Harrer, G., and Schulz, V., "Clinical investigation of the antidepressant effectiveness of hypericum," *Journal of Geriatric Psychiatry and Neurology* 7 suppl. 1 (1994) S6–8.

Harrer, G., and Sommer, H., "Treatment of mild/moderate depressions with hypericum," *Phytomedicine* 1/1 (1994) 3–8.

Hawken, C. M., *St. John's Wort* (Pleasant Grove, UT: Woodland Books, 1997).

Herbs for Health staff, "St. John's wort offers natural therapy," *Herbs for Health* 2/5 (Nov./Dec. 1997) 26–30.

Hobbs, C., "St. John's wort, *Hypericum perforatum*," *HerbalGram* 18/19 (1989) 24–33.

Hoffmann, D., *The New Holistic Herbal* (Rockport, ME: Element Books, 1992).

Holzl, J., "Inhaltestoffe und Wirkmechanismen des Johanniskrauts," *Zeiuchnfi fur Phytotherapie* 14 (1993) 255–64.

Hubner, W., Lande, S., and Podzuweit, H., "Hypericum treatment of mild depressions with somatic symptoms," *Journal of Geriatric Psychiatry and Neurology* 7 suppl. 1 (1994) S12–14.

Hudson, J. B., Harris, L., and Towers, G. H., "The importance of light in the anti-HIV effect of hypericin," *Antiviral Research* 20/2 (1993) 173–178.

Hudson, J. B., Lopez-Bazzocchi, I., and Towers, G., "Antiviral activities of hypericin," *Antiviral Research* 15/2 (1991) 101–112.

Hutchens, A., *A Handbook of Native American Herbs* (Boston: Shambhala, 1992).

James, J. S. "AIDS," *Treatment News* 117 (1990) 3.

———, "Hypericum: Common herb shows anti-retroviral activity," *AIDS Treatment News* (Aug. 26, 1988).

Jenike, M. A., "Hypericum: A novel antidepressant," *Journal of Geriatric Psychiatry and Neurology* 7 suppl. 1 (1994) S1.

Johnson, D., Siebenhunder, G., Hofer, E., et al., "Emflu[beta] von Johanniskraut auf die ZNS-Aktintat," *Neurologie/Psychiatrie* 6 (1992) 436–444.

Johnson, D., et al., "Effects of hypericum extract LI 160 compared with maprotiline on resting EEG and evoked potentials in 24 volunteers," *Journal of Geriatric Psychiatry and Neurology* 7 suppl. 1 (1994) S44–46.

Kugler, J., Weidenhammer, W., et al., "Therapie depressiver Zustande," *Zeichri fur Allgemeinmedizein* 66 (1990) 21–30.

Lavie, G., et al., "Hypericin as an inactivator of infectious viruses in blood components," *Transfusion* 35/5 (1995) 392–400.

Lee, P., "St. John's wort," *Total Health* 11/4 (1989) 33–35.

Lerhl, S., and Woelk, H., "Ergebnisse von Messungen der kognitiven Leistungsfahigkeit bei Patienten unter der therapie mit Johanniskraut," *Nevernheilkunde* 12 (1993) 281–285.

Linde, K., Ramirez, G., Mulrow, C. D., et al., "St. John's wort for depression—an overview and meta-analysis of randomized clinical trials," *British Medical Journal* 313/7052 (Aug. 3, 1996) 253–258.

Mars, B., "An herbalist's approach," *Herbs for Health* (Nov./Dec. 1996) 53.

Martinez, B., Kasper, S., Ruhrmann, S., and Moller, H. J., "Hypericum in the treatment of seasonal affective disorders," *Journal of Geriatric Psychiatry and Neurology* 7/1 (1994) 29–33.

Meruelo, D., Lavie, G., and Lavie, D., "Therapeutic agents with dramatic antiretroviral activity and little toxicity at effective doses: Aromatic polycyclic diones hypericin and pseudohypericin," *Proceedings of the National Academy of Sciences of the United States of America* 85/14 (1988) 5230–5234.

Miller, S., "St. John's wort: A natural mood booster," *Newsweek* (May 5, 1997).

Monmaney, T., "Herb may help ease depression," *Los Angeles Times* (Aug. 2, 1996).

Muldner, H., and Aoller, M., "Antidepressive effect of a hypericum extract standardized to an active hypericin complex: Biochemistry and clinical studies," *Arzeinmittelforschung* 34/8 (1984) 918–920.

Muller, W., and Rossol, R., "Effects of hypericum extract on the expression of serotonin receptors," *Journal of Geriatric Psychiatry and Neurology* 7/1 (1994) S63–64.

Nash, M. J., "Natural Prozac? Despite growing popularity, St. John's wort has yet to convince skeptics it is safe and effective," *Time* (Sept. 22, 1997).

Ody, P., *The Complete Medicinal Herbal* (London: Dorling Kindersley, 1993).

Osterheider, M., Schmidtke, A., and Beckmann, H., "Behandlung depressiver Syndrome mit Hypericum (Johanniskraut) eine placebokontrollierte Doppelblundstudie," *Foruchritre rler Neunologie/Psychiatrie* 60/ suppl. 2 (1992) 210–211.

Prevention editors, "St. John's wort," in *Healing Herbs* (Emmaus, PA: Rodale Press, 1996).

Quandt, J., Schmidt, U., and Schenk, N., "Ambuliante Behandlung leichter und mittelschwerer depressiver Versimmungen," *Der Allgemeinarzt* 2 (1993) 97102.

Reh, C., Laux, P., and Shenk, N., "Hypericum-Extrakt bei Depressionen—eine wirksame Alternative," *Therapiewoche* 42 (1992) 1576–1582.

Reichert, R., "St. John's wort extract as a tricyclic medication substitute for mild to moderate depression," *Quarterly Review of Natural Medicine* (Winter 1995) 275–278.

Schmidt, U., Harrer, G., Kuhn U., et al., "Wechselwirkungen von Hyper-icin-Extrakt mit Alkohol," *Nervenheilkunde* 12/3 (1993) 14–23.

Schmidt, U., and Sommer, H., "Johanniskraut-Extrakt zur ambulanten therapie der Depression," *Fortschritte Der Medizin* 111 (1993) 339–342.

Schulz, H., and Jobert, M., "Effects of hypericum extract on the sleep EEG in older volunteers," *Journal of Geriatric Psychiatry and Neurology* 7 suppl. 1 (1994) S39–43.

Seattle Treatment Education Project, "Hypericin: A fact sheet," *Seattle Treatment Education Project* (June 1996).

Shepherd, R. C. H., "A Canadian isolate of *Colletotrichum gloesporooides* as a potential biological control agent for St. John's wort in Australia," *Plant Protection Quarterly* 10/4 (1995) 148–151.

Someya, H., "Effect of constituent of *Hypericum-erectum* on infection and multiplication of Epstein-Barr virus," *Journal of Tokyo Medical College* 43/5 (1985) 815–826.

Sommer, H., and Harrer, G., "Placebo-controlled double-blind study examining the effectiveness of a hypericum preparation in 105 mildly depressed patients," *Journal of Geriatric Psychiatry and Neurology* 7 suppl. 1 (1994) S9–11.

Staffeldt, B., Kerb, R., et al., "Pharmacokinetics of hypericin and pseudohypericin after oral intake of the *Hypericum perforatum* extract LI 160 in healthy volunteers," *Journal of Geriatric Psychiatry and Neurology* 7 suppl. 1 (1994) S47–53.

Suzuki, O., et al., "Inhibition of monoamine oxidase by hypericin," *Planta Medica* (1984) 272–274.

Tenney, L., *Today's Herbal Health* (Pleasant Grove, UT: Woodland Books, 1992).

Thiele, B., Brink, I., and Ploch, M., "Modulation of cytokine expression by hypericum extract," *Journal of Geriatric Psychiatry and Neurology* 7 suppl. 1 (1994) S60–62.

Thiele, H. M., and Walper, A., "Inhibition of MAO and COMT by hypericum extracts and hypericin," *Journal of Geriatric Psychiatry and Neurology* 7 suppl. 1 (1994) S54–56.

Tierra, L., *The Herbs of Life* (Freedom, CA: Crossing Press, 1992).

Tilford, G., "St. John's wort," *Natural Pet Magazine* (Sept./Oct. 1997) 33–39.

Tyler, V. E., *Herbs of Choice: The Therapeutic Use of Phytomedicinals* (London: Haworth Press, 1994).

———, "St. John's wort: The leading herb for mild to moderate depression," *Natural Pharmacy* 1/2 (Feb. 1997) 8.

Vorbach, E., Hubner, W., and Arnoldt, K., "Effectiveness and tolerance of the hypericum extract LI 160 compared to imipramine: Randomized double blind study with 135 outpatients," *Journal of Geriatric Psychiatry and Neurology* 7 suppl. 1 (1994) S19–23.

Wagner, H., and Bladt, S., "Pharmaceutical quality of hypericum extracts," *Journal of Geriatric Psychiatry and Neurology* 7 suppl. 1 (1994) S65–68.

Weiner, M., *Weiner's Herbal* (Mill Valley, CA: Quantum Books, 1990).

Weiner, M., and Weiner, J., *Herbs That Heal: Prescription for Herbal Healing* (Mill Valley, CA: Quantum Books, 1994).

Weiser, D., "Pharmacokinetics of hypericin after oral administration of St. John's extract," *Nerverheilkunde* 10/7 (1991) A17–18.

Willard, T., *The Wild Rose Scientific Herbal* (Calgary, Alberta: Wild Rose College of Natural Healing, 1991).

Witte, B., Harrer, G., Kaptan, T., Podzuweit, H., and Schmidt, U., "Behandlung depressiver Verstimmungen mit einem hochkonzentrierten

Hypercumpraparat; Eine multizentrische plazebocontrollierte Doppelblind-studie," *Fortschritte Der Medizin* 113 (1995) 46–54.

Woelk, H., Burkard, G., and Grunwald, J., "Benefits and risk of the hypericum extract LI 160: Drug monitoring study with 3250 patients," *Journal of Geriatric Psychiatry and Neurology* 7 suppl. 1 (1994) S34–8.

Yip, L., et al., "Antiviral activity of a derivative of the photosensitive compound hypericin," *Phytomedicine* 3/2 (1996) 185–190.

Index

DUE DATE			
⑦ SEP 1 5 1998		4DEC 1 5 1998